# Communicating with Vulnerable Children

# Communicating with Vulnerable Children

## A Guide for Practitioners

David P. H. Jones

Gaskell

Gaskell is an imprint of the Royal College of Psychiatrists, 17 Belgrave Square,
London SW1X 8PG, UK
http://www.rcpsych.ac.uk

British Library Cataloguing-in-Publication Data
A catalogue record for this book is available from the British Library.
ISBN 1-901242-91-9

Distributed in North America by Balogh International Inc.

The views presented in this book do not necessarily reflect those of the Royal
College of Psychiatrists, and the publishers are not responsible for any error of
omission or fact.

The Royal College of Psychiatrists is a registered charity (no. 228636).

Printed in Great Britain by Bell & Bain Limited, Thornliebank, Glasgow.

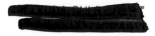

# Contents

*List of boxes, tables and figures*     viii
*Acknowledgements*     x
*Copying of material from this book*     xii
*Foreword*     xiii
*Preface*     xv

1   Introduction and orientation     1
     Organisation and suggested use

**Part I. The knowledge base**
2   Developmental considerations     9
     General understanding
     Memory
     Suggestibility
     The consistency of children's recall over time
     Language development
     Social and emotional development
     Conclusions

3   Erroneous concerns and cases     33
     Terminology
     The consequences of erroneous concern
     Frequency of types of false positive errors
     Mechanisms leading to false positive cases of abuse

4   The child's psychological condition     38
     The effects of adverse experiences on children
     Some special problems
     The effect of the child's psychological condition on communication

5   Diversity and difference: implications for practice     49
     Race, culture and language
     Disabled children

6   Successful communication: core skills and basic principles     64
     Self-management
     Technique
     Implications for the practitioner
     Summary

7   How concerns come to professional attention:
    the context for practice                                                    73
        Use and misuse of the term 'disclosure'
        Developmental considerations
        Social and emotional factors
        Children at different stages in the child protection system
        Children's presentations of sexual abuse allegations
        Children's accounts subsequent to discovery of physical harm
        Qualitative studies of children's experiences of telling others
        Adult recollections of childhood abuse
        Delay in disclosing adverse experiences
        Have sexual assault prevention programmes affected the presentation
            of concerns?
        Summary

Part II. Practice issues
8   Practice issues: introduction                                              87

9   Talking with the child: first responses to children's
    concerns                                                                    91
        Policy and procedural issues
        Research findings concerning first responses
        Implications for practitioners

10  Talking with children about adverse events during
    initial assessments                                                        101
        The policy and procedural context
        Research findings
        Implications for practitioners
        Summary

11  In-depth interviews with children                                         114
        The policy and procedural context
        Research findings and practice implications
        A schema for undertaking in-depth interviews

12  Indirect and non-verbal approaches                                        145
        Observation
        Toys and drawings
        Research findings
        Implications for practitioners

13  Advice for parents and carers                                             157
        First concerns
        Advice during the process of assessment
        When uncertainty persists

14   Epilogue                                                    162
        A framework for analysis
        Training
        Future directions for practice development

     References                                                  173

     Index                                                       183

# Boxes, tables and figures

**Boxes**
2.1  Developmental changes in children's understanding     10
2.2  Circumstances in which children are especially
     susceptible to suggestion     18
4.1  Possible effects of domestic violence upon children     41
5.1  Consequences of a child's impairment that present
     challenges for practitioners     61
5.2  Good practice at the organisational planning level     62
5.3  Good practice for individual practitioners     63
6.1  Core skills and qualities professionals need to
     communicate effectively with children     65
9.1  Summary of first responses to children's concerns
     expressed to front-line practitioners     100
10.1 Exploratory questions     110
11.1 Occasions when professionals other than social workers
     undertake in-depth interviews     115
11.2 Principal issues for practitioners undertaking in-depth
     interviews     116
11.3 Summary of the principal findings relating to the accuracy
     of children's accounts of adverse events     118
11.4 Obtaining reliable accounts     119
11.5 Items to consider when planning an in-depth interview     122
11.6 Possible areas to cover with the child in preparation for
     an in-depth interview     124
11.7 Summary of the principal implications from research for
     practitioners undertaking in-depth interviews     129
11.8 Prompts and questions to direct a child's attention to
     issues of concern     131
11.9 Communicating with children when interviews end in
     uncertainty     139
12.1 A schema for describing observations of behaviour     146
12.2 Issues involving the use of toys, drawings and props in
     interviews     149
12.3 Summary practice points for the use of toys, drawing
     and props     156
13.1 Advice professionals can give to parents who are concerned
     their child may have been harmed or traumatised     158

13.2  Ingredients of parent preparation                          160
13.3  Advice for parents, in uncertain circumstances            161

**Tables**
3.1  Mechanisms through which erroneous cases occur           36
4.1  Psychological impairments and problems associated
       with childhood abuse                                      40

**Figure**
8.1  The assessment process and different kinds of
       communication with children                              89

# Acknowledgements

## Department of Health Advisory Group

Ms Jenny Gray, Children's Services, Department of Health, London (Chair)

Dr Jan Aldridge, Senior Lecturer in Clinical Psychology, University of Leeds

Mr Simon Barter, Thames Valley Police, Oxford

Ms Willma Bartlett, National Training and Development Officer, NSPCC, Leicester

Dr Arnon Bentovim, London Child and Family Clinic

Detective Chief Inspector Lynn Bowler, Derbyshire Constabulary

Professor Ray Bull, Department of Psychology, University of Portsmouth

Inspector Ian Clarke, Gloucestershire Constabulary

Professor Graham Davies, Department of Psychology, University of Leicester

Ms Maria Godfrey, Unit Manager, Children and Family Assessment Team, Oxfordshire Social Services Department

Ms Gillian Harrison, Home Office, London

David Holmes, Social Care Group 3, Department of Health, London

Dr Robert Jezzard, Senior Policy Advisor, Department of Health, London

Dr Helen Jones, Department of Health, London

Dr Caroline Lindsey, Royal College of Psychiatrists, London

Detective Sergeant Brian McDaid, Thames Valley Police, Reading

Ms Katrina McNamara, Department of Health, London

Detective Inspector John Meredith, Child Protection Unit, Thames Valley Police, Oxford

Ms Lorraine Morris, Pupil Support and Independent Schools Division, Department for Education and Skills, London

Mr Marcus Page, Triangle, Brighton, Sussex

Judge Isobel Plumstead QC, Principal Registry of the Family Division, London

Mr Aaran Poyser, Department of Health, London

Ms Gretchen Precey, Triangle, Brighton, Sussex

Detective Inspector Paul Purnell, Child Protection Unit, Gloucestershire Constabulary

Mr Dave Seal, Principal Officer, Child Protection, Oxfordshire Social Services Department

Mr Peter Smith, Department of Health, London

Ms Gail Treml, Department for Education and Skills, London

Dr Helen Westcott, Department of Psychology, Faculty of Social Sciences, The Open University

Mr Richard White, Solicitor, Croydon

Ms Sally Whitehouse, Child Protection Unit, Derbyshire Constabulary

## President's Interdisciplinary Committee, Advisory Group

The Right Honourable Lord Justice Matthew Thorpe, Royal Courts of Justice, London (Chair)

Ms Tess Duncan, Children's Guardian, Surrey

Dr Danya Glaser, Consultant Child and Adolescent Psychiatrist, Great Ormond Street Hospital for Children, London

Ms Jenny Kenrick, Consultant Child Psychotherapist, Tavistock Clinic, London

Dr Claire Sturge, Consultant Child Psychiatrist, Northwick Park Hospital, London

Dr Judith Trowell, Consultant Child and Adolescent Psychiatrist, Tavistock Clinic, London

The Honourable Mr Justice Nicholas Wall, Royal Courts of Justice, London

# Copying of material from this book

Permission from the publisher is not required when parts of individual chapters of this book are photocopied for the personal use of professionals working with vulnerable children. The statement of the source of the material must be preserved on any copies used. For reproduction of whole chapters, or of any part of this book for commercial purposes or on a website, written permission from the publishers is required.

# Foreword

My involvement in this wonderful book had its origins at a memorable conference convened at Satra Bruk in Sweden by Professor Michael Lamb, from the National Institute for Child Health and Development, Washington. Experts had been invited from Sweden, the United States, Israel and the United Kingdom to focus on methods of eliciting from child victims evidence of sufficient clarity and cogency to advance the prosecution of an adult abuser at a criminal trial. Our discussions also covered the extent to which professionals in the family justice system strained the Memorandum Guide (Home Office & Department of Health, 1992) to perform tasks that it was never designed to perform. We identified the obvious need for someone to prepare a bespoke guide for family justice, written by a family justice specialist for use by any professional in the context of family proceedings. Unbeknown to me, at that time the Department of Health was also having discussions about commissioning an evidence-based publication that would assist practitioners in their communications with vulnerable children. David Jones was approached because of his long experience and special interest in interviewing children.

The subsequent development of this book has been guided by an advisory group convened by the Department of Health. The President's Interdisciplinary Committee has furnished additional support by reading and commenting upon the developing draft. What has emerged will, I am confident, be received with wide acclaim throughout the family justice system. It meets a crucial need. Its division into a review of the knowledge base followed by the essential guidance on practice issues confirms the scholarship and scientific knowledge by which the reader is guided. The division of the readership into various professional categories with a suggested reading list appropriate for each makes the journey into the text immediately inviting and destroys any fear that the reader will be overwhelmed. Of course the guide is not written with judges particularly in mind, but I suggest that we would all benefit from a selective reading of this masterly summary of available research and good practice.

The publication of this new and vital book has been supported throughout by the Department of Health. I commend it to the specialist judges, barristers and solicitors in the Family Justice system as an authoritative practice resource. It is my hope that this new and vital book will be not in the library but at the fingertips of all who regularly work with vulnerable children.

*the Right Honourable Lord Justice Thorpe*

# Preface

This book is about much more than talking. Communication is a two-way process. Being receptive, through listening, hearing or alternative means, is a necessary precondition, while during our attempts to communicate, so much is transmitted between us non-verbally. Even when words can be found, we convey meaning through reliance on inflection, timing and accompanying gesture, along with words themselves. For some children other forms of language are preferred, for example sign or other means of augmentative communication. Hence, although we think of 'talking' with children, the term 'communication' is used liberally throughout the book, in order to emphasise the range of activities involved in sharing, imparting, transmitting, and receiving information between children and adults.

Effective communicating is a central part of the work with children and their parents that is brought into sharp relief when children have adverse experiences they want to talk about. This book has arisen from considering the challenges involved in talking with children in these circumstances. Its aim is to set out the research and evidence base on communicating with children in an accessible form and to provide suggestions for effective practice.

I was guided by many in this task, but mostly by the experience of talking with children and young people and, occasionally, to adults reflecting and looking back on their childhood. Accurate accounts are an essential basis for effective care planning and psychological treatment. My experiences within American and English family courts also underlined how important it was to obtain as full and accurate an understanding as possible about what children were trying to communicate, and I am grateful to those who work within the family courts for raising the critical issues. Many other colleagues in a wide variety of professions have influenced and shaped the practice guidance expressed in this book. They come from child and family mental health, adult mental health, social work with children and families, police investigators within child protection units, education services and within the field of experimental psychology, among other disciplines. These colleagues have provided essential questions, thoughts, advice, stimulation and challenge. I thank them all, in the USA, the UK and Europe.

The work behind this book was only possible because the Department of Health in England provided a grant to release me from clinical work for four months, in order to start the process of analysing the evidence base. I am also indebted to my colleagues at the Park Hospital, and the Oxfordshire Mental Healthcare NHS Trust, who not only agreed for me to undertake this work, but lent support and encouragement too.

The Department of Health set up an expert advisory group who went over every idea and statement in this book, challenging them and constructively criticising the work as it evolved. I want to thank each of them for their help. Their names are listed in the Acknowledgements. Similarly, the President's Interdisciplinary Committee from the Family Division of the High Court of Justice read and critiqued early drafts, also helping to mould the final product. The advisory group's comments and support throughout have been of enormous value. Readers from that committee are also listed in the Acknowledgements. Lord Justice Mathew Thorpe chaired the advisory group, but also consistently encouraged me in the project from start to finish and kept a steady eye on the final goal. I wish also to thank Professor Michael Lamb of the National Institute for Child Health and Human Development, Washington, DC, for his insightful comments and advice on the first draft and for his ongoing interest and support in this venture.

The project was commissioned and then expertly guided by Jenny Gray from the Children's Services Section of the Department of Health. I am especially grateful to her and her Section for consistent support, advice and encouragement, as well as meticulous editing of my ideas as they evolved throughout the life of this project. Her comprehensive appreciation of the field and all the different practitioners who work with children has been of inestimable value throughout this project.

*D.P.H.J., Oxford, November 2002*

# CHAPTER 1

# Introduction and orientation

This book is designed to help those who seek to communicate with children who may have had personally adverse or sensitive experiences. It is primarily orientated towards front-line practitioners such as social workers, teachers, children's guardians and child mental health professionals. The central focus of the book is on facilitating the child's welfare rather than obtaining information for other purposes, such as criminal prosecution.

Many professionals communicate with children and young people each day as an integral part of their job. The vast majority of these contacts are unconnected with adversity, but purposeful and governed by the nature of the professional's job. For example, teachers, health visitors and youth workers cover a wide range of children's experiences during the course of their everyday work. Sometimes, sensitive or traumatic issues enter these exchanges, especially when they have been part of the child's life and experiences. However, for other professionals (e.g. social workers, psychologists and psychiatrists), communication about distress and confusion is a major component of their work. This book emerged from the perceived need for these various types of communication to be described and the methods used by professionals in these different circumstances to be critically reviewed, in order to gather together good practice recommendations. It is orientated towards the needs of professionals who work directly with children, whether they are generalists or provide specialist services, but where the welfare of the child becomes a matter for concern. Welfare itself is a broad concept and includes physical and mental health, safety and freedom from harm or abuse, together with children's rights to express themselves and to be heard, as well as to be involved in matters that will affect them (de Mello, 2000).

Professionals require the means to communicate effectively with children and young people who are in a wide variety of situations. They therefore need to discover ways of communicating with children who find it difficult to do so because of their age, an impairment or their particular psychological or social situation. Professionals must ensure that any accounts of adverse experiences coming from children are as accurate and complete as possible. Accuracy is key, for without it effective decisions cannot be made and, equally, inaccurate accounts can lead to children remaining unsafe, or to the possibility of wrongful

Source: Jones, D. P. H. (2003) *Talking with Vulnerable Children*. London: Gaskell.

actions being taken that affect children and adults. Similarly, incomplete accounts are also problematic. Fundamentally, inaccurate and/or incomplete accounts fail children who have experienced adversity, as well as those who in fact have not, but where a professional thinks they may have been. This is because children's accounts influence decision making in a number of different arenas. Examples include decisions that may be made about their own welfare (including, but not limited to, protection issues), and those made about children's residence or their contact with family or others. This book draws together available evidence in order to inform practice, training and supervision.

When concerns about a child's welfare first emerge, it is often not possible to predict where they will lead. For instance, it cannot always be predicted whether the child's first communications will eventually result in significant child welfare decisions, family justice orders, criminal justice action and prosecution of an offender, or merely no further action being required. Nonetheless, the guiding premise here is that all children, regardless of their personal and social situation, should be provided with the best opportunity to communicate any concerns they may have. The book is not a blueprint for all communications or interviews with children. Interviewing children is a difficult task, and each child is unique. However, the principles set out here are intended as pointers to good practice, based upon the present state of knowledge in the field. This is considered from the point of view of what scientific evidence there is concerning different types of communication strategies in relation to accuracy and completeness of accounts, and, where scientific evidence is not available, the advice in this guide will be based on consensus. Sometimes, however, neither scientific evidence nor consensus is available, and in these circumstances the different choices facing the interviewer will be set out.

## Organisation and suggested use

The book is divided into two main parts: I, The knowledge base (Chapters 2–7); and II, Practice issues (Chapters 8–13). Part I provides overviews of those areas that are especially important for those communicating with children. Each chapter contains summaries of key points, and the implications for practitioners that emerge at strategic points.

Part II begins with a chapter describing the various situations in which professionals may be required to hear children's concerns. In Chapter 9 considers practice when concerns emerge during the course of a professional's everyday activities. The next two chapters provide an increasingly explicit focus on assessing the welfare status of the child. Indirect and non-verbal approaches are discussed in Chapter 12. Advice for parents is set out in Chapter 13.

Jones, D. P. H. (2003) *Communicating with Vulnerable Children*. London: Gaskell.

Finally, an epilogue presents a framework for the analysis of children's disclosures and points out the need for training in this area. Some future directions for research are suggested.

This book is intended to be of value to a wide range of professionals who work with children. Some readers will only need selected chapters or summaries, while others may find more sections useful to their practice. The following suggestions are intended to lead the reader rapidly to those sections that are likely to prove most relevant to their work with children and families, although it is recommended that readers first use the remainder of this chapter to orientate themselves to this book's relationship to national guidance and policy.

**Professionals providing an everyday service which all, or many, children receive, such as primary health care, education or social care (e.g. teachers, health visitors, youth workers, residential social workers).**

Start with Chapter 8, followed by the implications for practitioners on pages 53–55, and the summaries in Box 5.1 (p. 61), and Box 5.3 (p. 63). Then read Chapter 9, particularly the implications for practitioners starting at page 97 and summarised in Box 9.1 (p. 100).

**Professionals whose role occasionally includes concern about whether a child has suffered adversity (e.g. designated teachers, paediatricians, community child health workers and child and adolescent mental health service workers)**

Similarly to the first group of professionals, start with Chapter 8, followed by the implications for practitioners on pages 53–55, and the summaries in Box 5.1 (p. 61) and Box 5.3 (p. 63). Then read Chapter 9, particularly the implications for practitioners starting at page 97, and summarised in Box 9.1 (p. 100). If you wish to provide advice for parents, this is summarised in Box 13.1 (p. 158). Then read Chapters 7 and 10. Summaries of key points appear on pages 81–83, 112–113, and in Box 10.1 (p. 111).

**Professionals who are especially concerned with assessing a child's needs, including where there may be concerns about possible harm (e.g., specialist social workers undertaking core assessments as part of Section 47 enquiries under the Children Act; other professionals who may be undertaking similar assessment interviews, or assisting social workers to undertake Section 47 enquiries; children's guardians, children and family reporters, and lawyers and judges in the family justice system)**

While it is anticipated that the whole text will be of value, these professionals may wish to follow the sequence recommended immediately above, before reviewing Chapters 11 and 12.

Jones, D. P. H. (2003) *Communicating with Vulnerable Children*. London: Gaskell.

3

## Links with government policy and professional guidance

This book's purpose is to identify best practice in a difficult area of work. It is a practice resource, based upon the best evidence available: it is not statutory guidance.

Government guidance on what to do if a professional considers a child to be in need is clearly set out in the *Framework for the Assessment of Children in Need and Their Families* (Department of Health *et al*, 2000; National Assembly for Wales, 2001). *Working Together to Safeguard Children: A Guide to Inter-agency Working to Safeguard and Promote the Welfare of Children* (Department of Health *et al*, 1999, especially paras 5.5. and 5.6; National Assembly for Wales, 2000) is the government's guidance for those working with a child who is, or may be, suffering significant harm. This may result in Section 47 enquiries, led by social workers, in order to ascertain whether a child is suffering or likely to suffer significant harm. If it is considered that a child may have been the subject of a criminal offence, then the police should be involved in investigating a possible crime. They, together with the social services department plus other agencies, should also consider how best to safeguard the individual child. Sometimes this will involve the need for an investigative interview to gather evidence for criminal proceedings. *Achieving Best Evidence* (Home Office *et al*, 2002) is the recognised good practice guide for all videotaped, investigative interviews with children, for this latter purpose.

## Areas of work to which this book will apply

The above is a very brief summary of the framework within which professionals in England and Wales operate when there are concerns that a child is or may be suffering harm, or a crime is thought to have been committed. There are many situations where concerns exist about a child's welfare but the situation is not yet well defined. This publication brings together principles and practice about communication with children in these less-well-defined situations, within the overall framework set out in the government's guidance. Some examples of these less-well-defined situations follow.

A 12-year-old black boy tells his teacher that he does not want to go home. It is not clear why, but he has previously indicated that all is not well in his foster home. He has seemed unhappy in school, his schoolwork has worsened and he appears to have few friends, especially during the past three months. How can the teacher respond to this boy's expressed reluctance to go home?

A white girl aged six years has been referred to the local social services department by her school because of long-standing concerns about neglect. These concerns have now been heightened by the finding of two small bruises on the left side of her face, combined with the teacher's growing unease about the child's predicament. The social worker arrives to see the child. The social worker's first objective is to communicate with the child to try to assess whether it is safe for her to go home, and, if it is, whether any other services or assessments be initiated.

A ten-year-old white girl has talked to her mother about having been sexually assaulted by her father, who had left the family home approximately two months before. She has pleaded with her mother not to tell anyone. Her mother telephones the social services department, uncertain what to do next. The social worker's first contact with the child is to ascertain whether she is willing and able to communicate her concerns to professional staff.

A 14-year-old white boy has been picked up by the police in the centre of a small town, having drunk excess alcohol and taken illicit drugs. He has not attended school for several months and spends much of the day in the house of a man in his thirties, where several disaffected local young people spend their daytimes and evenings. The 14-year-old describes pornographic activities. He is vague about his own level of involvement, but names three other young people. How should these other three be first approached? And what principles and communication practices might assist?

Further examples of the area of work for which this book is intended include those children who have been witness to domestic violence within their households (and domestic violence may involve serious assault by one member of the household on another and even murder). Such children may have been through criminal investigations or Section 47 enquiries (or both) but may now reside in foster care, where new but relatively non-specific concerns arise. Concerns about children's welfare arise in many other contexts, too such as child referrals to mental health services, or those involved in court welfare services, or where children's guardians have the task of assessing a child's views, wishes or feelings about specific people or issues.

Where a crime may have been committed, it is not always possible to know at the outset whether the case will unfold in the direction of major social work or police investigations, or a combination of the two. Much depends on what the child has to say initially. For this reason the secondary aim of this book is to ensure that these first approaches to children by professionals do not compromise future assessments or investigations, should these eventually prove necessary. Thus professionals should always be aware of the necessity of referral to specialist assessment and police investigation services at any time during the unfolding of a child's concerns.

There are many cases that fall short of those that warrant referral to a specialist assessment service, as well as children and young people who have already been subject to police investigations that have led to inconclusive outcomes but where generalised concerns continue nonetheless. This book is intended to be of assistance in a wide range of situations and sets out background principles and a practical approach to children and young people, whatever the nature of the case.

Different professions have their own literature describing good practice with respect to the assessment of children. The present book is intended to supplement rather than replace these resources.

Jones, D. P. H. (2003) *Communicating with Vulnerable Children*. London: Gaskell.

# Part I

# The knowledge base

---

The chapters in Part I contain overviews of topics that are particularly important to those communicating with children who may have suffered harm. The chapters highlight important areas of concern for practitioners and refer interested readers to further texts for comprehensive coverage of each topic. Summaries of practice implications are contained within, or at the end of, each chapter.

# CHAPTER 2

# Developmental considerations

Sensitivity to children's development is an essential skill for all those working with children and young people. Development involves the relatively ordered and lasting changes that occur over time in the person's physical structure, thought processes, behaviour and emotions. During the course of childhood there are major psychological and psychosocial changes as the child becomes more organised, competent and also more complex. There is agreement among researchers and theorists that the key stages involve: early attachment to a carer (or carers) in the first 12 months of life; a period of self-development (up to the age of three years); a period in which relationships with other children become key (ages three to seven years); and, following this, the integration of attachment, self-development and peer relationships (up to adolescence) (Cicchetti, 1989; Masten & Coatsworth, 1998).

In this chapter we will note selected developmental issues of special importance when a professional communicates with traumatised or maltreated children. First, though, a warning is needed concerning ideas about children's development. Great care should be exercised when considering the expected developmental stages and the ages at which they occur. This information is generally presented in books and training packs according to the usual course of development for most children. These present a useful framework and provide a guide for professionals (for a general introduction see Daniel *et al*, 1999). However, there is enormous variation between children, created by genetic factors as well as environmental influences. Thus all the comments made below concerning typical ages at which children achieve certain competencies must be taken as general markers, which may require adapting to the individual child. Further, much of what follows concerns children who have not been maltreated. We now know that living in an abusive environment significantly alters the progress and pattern of children's development (see Chapter 4).

The area of developmental psychology and its application to forensic and child welfare practice is vast. Listed in this chapter are the most important findings relevant to communicating with children and their practice implications. More detailed reviews and commentaries are available in Ceci & Bruck (1995), Poole & Lamb (1998) and Westcott *et al* (2002). The following areas are covered here: children's general understanding, memory, suggestibility, language, and social and

---

**Box 2.1** Developmental changes in children's understanding

- Children's general knowledge about the world is limited by experience.
- The ability to appreciate the nature of other people's attitudes, thoughts and feelings, and to understand that these may differ from one's own, comes in later childhood.
- Older children and adolescents have their expectations shaped by prior experience. They may therefore have fixed expectations about how people in authority might react to them (e.g. black teenagers' expectations of the police).
- Younger children have not necessarily considered the consequences of describing adverse experiences to others. Older children may well have done so, or have attitudes already shaped by their own or others' experiences.

---

emotional development. The intent is to stimulate the reader further by setting out the main areas that have salience for practitioners. The danger of this selective approach is reductionism. However, it is hoped that in stressing the wide variation and extensive individual differences, readers will be made more curious rather than have their horizons restricted.

# General understanding

The first and most significant developmental change is an obvious one: the child's understanding and knowledge of the world expands rapidly during childhood. The pre-school child's world is a relatively narrow one, inhabited by immediate carers and a small number of friends. Knowledge about other people and their thoughts or intentions, both in general as well as knowledge about violence or sexual matters, is likely to be limited. This knowledge and social competence increases rapidly from the of age three years onwards and particularly during the school years (see Box 2.1). Hence a young child's understanding of events is likely to be significantly different from an adult perspective. One can often see this mismatch in the conversations between adults and younger children. Perhaps the overriding issue for professionals is one of being constantly alert to this difference, which will lead interviewers to check and review their understanding of the child's communications (see Chapter 6).

# Memory

A child's or adult's memory about an event is not akin to a videotape, residing somewhere in the individual's mind which, if only it were to be connected to an appropriate machine, could be successfully replayed. Memory is not 'hard-wired' but is instead a much more malleable set of systems and processes, which are affected by circumstances at the time of an event occurring, as well as the mental processing that occurs in the interim and at the time of recall. An understanding of these fundamental aspects of human memory is essential for practice when communicating effectively with children.

The following represents a brief overview of selected aspects of memory that are relevant for the practitioner. General accounts of memory development can be found in textbooks of infant and child development (e.g. Atkinson *et al*, 1996; Mussen *et al*, 1990, pp. 115–121, 314–323, 582; Bornstein & Lamb, 1992, pp. 279–287). Summaries of aspects relevant to practice with vulnerable children include Ceci and Bruck (1995), Poole & Lamb (1998) and Westcott *et al* (2002). For more detailed reviews of children's memory for events, see Conway (1996), Howe & Courage (1997), Wheeler *et al* (1997), Gathercole (1998) and Siegel (2001).

Memory can be defined as the process of storing what is attended to, and then being able to retrieve and use that information (Bornstein & Lamb, 1992). Memory lies at the heart of the developing child's learning, understanding and capacity to use language to communicate with others. As we have already noted, it is not a single entity but is better thought of as a collection of systems and processes which allow a person to retrieve the past and make use of this for present action and planning what to do next. Thus, memory can be thought of as describing the mechanisms through which past events affect future functioning.

There are several different ways of understanding and thinking about this collection of systems and processes that we call memory. A great deal depends upon the frame of reference being considered and the purpose of any distinctions being made. For example, when we are considering the timing of memory processes and stages, it is useful to distinguish sensory memory (also called the 'sensory register') from short-term and long-term memory. Alternatively, distinctions can be made between remembering 'about' things (declarative memory) and remembering 'how to do' a thing (procedural memory). Remembering about things is often divided into semantic and episodic memory. All these are discussed in more detail below.

We can also think about memory in terms of its content, and for our purposes we are especially interested in autobiographical memory and event memory. However, practitioners are also concerned about changes in children's abilities as they grow and develop. We now understand that it is the child's performance that alters significantly over time, rather than structural changes within the brain. Hence, children's capacity to retrieve information from memory and convey this to others, while at the same time relating such memories to themselves, develops apace after approximately the age of two years. Not only does language improve but the child's ability both to retain and to retrieve memories does too. Children learn tricks and the best methods for remembering information. We learn these techniques as young children from those around us, as well as from our own experiences of remembering and forgetting (see Howe & Courage, 1997; Wheeler *et al*, 1997).

Notwithstanding these difficulties in conceptualising and defining memory, some distinctions are likely to be helpful for the practitioner and are briefly reviewed now. From a temporal perspective, three different types of memory can be distinguished, sensory memory, short-term memory and long-term memory. Sensory memory is the most brief and refers to the temporary storage of that which is attended to. Unless it is stored it will be forgotten in less than a second. Short-term memory is sometimes called working memory, and allows us to hold information just seen or heard for about 30 seconds (e.g. remembering a telephone number for just long enough to dial it). This working memory refers to how children and adults filter and retain information that they have received from the world around them, in verbal or visual form (Gathercole, 1998).

Long-term memory, sometimes called permanent memory, is what usually coincides with the lay use of the word memory. It describes our permanent storehouse of knowledge and information (e.g. repeating the same telephone number enough times, or with added tags of information so that it is distinctive, so that we can remember it for a long period).

There are two broad types of long-term memory, semantic and episodic. Semantic memory principally concerns facts and those things we simply 'know' about the world, which have built up over time. It includes our memory for words and our knowledge of names, places and faces. We usually do not remember when we learnt these aspects of semantic knowledge but we just 'know' that we know them. Semantic memory can be thought of as the individual's internal reference library, which has been built up from their experience and evolving knowledge about the world.

Episodic memory is our memory for particular episodes and events that we have experienced. Some authorities consider episodic and autobiographical memory to be synonymous. Others confine episodic memory to our memory of events that took place relatively recently, perhaps during the past few days. Additionally, these authors restrict the term to those events of low personal salience or relevance (Conway, 1996; Gathercole, 1998). Such episodic memories are considered distinct from autobiographical memories, which are memories of events and classes of events remembered over much longer periods – weeks, months, or sometimes for many years. Such events are usually personally salient and the memory itself is accompanied by the memory of oneself in relation to the events being recalled. There are different types of autobiographical memory knowledge: memories of specific events, general groupings or classes of events (e.g. memory of going to a particular school each morning) and memories of sections or areas of one's life (e.g. 'the time I lived in South London'). When we remember events that are stored in our autobiographical memory system we draw upon each of these tiers of knowledge in order to bring out a single memory. Other authorities combine episodic and autobiographical memory and simply draw attention to the fact that autobiographical memory begins to appear only in the pre-school years, somewhere between the ages of two and four years.

## Memory stages: encoding, storage and retrieval

Memory can be broadly considered to involve three main stages: encoding (registering), storage (committing memory of events to either short-term or long-term storage) and retrieval (the act of recalling the past and remembering one's experiences). All three phases are affected by the state and circumstances of the individual at the time. Even if events are successfully encoded, subsequent experiences may still affect stored representations of events that are located in memory.

What is *encoded* or registered varies between individuals and also varies with age. Younger children's capacity to encode is less well formed and more likely to be idiosyncratic compared with that of older children and adults. This is partly because older children's overall knowledge of the world is greater and they know what to expect from situations.

Younger children, particularly those below the age of three, have significant difficulties in *retrieval*, particularly when asked to distinguish the source of a particular memory (so-called source-monitoring difficulties). With particularly demanding tasks, however, even older children and adults have similar difficulties. Younger children also have greater difficulty producing a narrative account of an event, even if they are capable of recalling it.

What is registered or encoded is always less than the total amount that could be remembered about a particular situation. How much is remembered depends upon the individual's interest, the salience or relevance of the event and other factors such as stress and the influence of other competing events at the time. Stress probably negatively affects an individual's ability to encode and store information accurately. However, emotionally laden events (both positive and negative) can be accurately recalled even after long periods of time.

The strength of memory that is *stored* varies according to: what seems to the person to be important or relevant; the amount of exposure to the event; and prior knowledge about similar matters. Younger children have less capacity to store information than older children. Moreover, if the memory is weak it is more susceptible to the effects of suggestion later on.

The *status* of memory changes over time. Younger children forget at a faster rate than older children and adults. Stored memory is also affected by subsequent events. If the memory is refreshed through rehearsal or discussion with others, it is more likely to be stored for longer. Equally, a child's own experiences of a similar type have an effect on any memory for a discrete event, moulding it and altering it.

*Retrieval* is similarly influenced by the state of the individual child and his or her psychological and social circumstances. The context in which retrieval occurs is very important. More distant memories are especially prone to suggestion at the point of retrieval and this has major implications for interviewing practice. However, those events that are highly significant or personally salient have been found to be relatively more resistant to suggestion than less personally important, 'peripheral' memories. In addition, those memories that are retrieved via free recall are more accurate than those retrieved via recognition (hence the superiority of more open questioning). When children remember past events actively they are using *recall*. However, when they are asked a leading question, that is, one that contains within it the answer that the practitioner suspects, the child 'remembers' by *recognising* whether the information provided is true or not. Not surprisingly, recall remembering is more accurate than recognition. Therefore, this is what practitioners should be aiming for (Lamb *et al*, 1999).

## The development of autobiographical memory

Children cannot usually remember events that happened in the first year of life. At least, they cannot do so verbally later on, even if those experiences have influenced the child's development. In the second year of life, sometimes children can remember events if they are put back in the same situation in which the events actually occurred. However, it is not until around 20 months that children first start to be able to talk about events that they have experienced. At first this is limited and usually dependent on being in the same situation in which the events occurred. During the third year of life they can recall events from several months previously, relatively freely. Younger children need questions from an adult to be able to do this, however. Children's accounts become progressively more detailed throughout the pre-school years. Provided questions are open ended, children's recall of past events during the pre-school years can be accurate. However, they frequently describe different aspects of the same experience as they grow older, presumably because their knowledge of the world is increasing rapidly, as well as their verbal capacity to convey their memories. Hence, inconsistency does not necessarily mean that children under six are inaccurate. The caveat, however, is that if questions are specific, or worse still misleading, young children's new information at progressive interviews is more likely to be in error (unlike the information that is repeated across interviews).

Single, isolated events, especially those that are distinctive, are more likely to be recalled in specific detail by children than those that are repeated every day or recurring events. Repeated events tend to get remembered as regular 'schemas' or 'script' memories, containing what usually happens, but unfortunately the memory for specific times or occasions seems to become somewhat submerged. This poses a major problem for practitioners who are talking with children about regular, repeated events, such as inter-parental conflict within the home. In these circumstances children will tend to describe what 'normally' happened, rather than relaying a specific occasion. We then have to find ways of linking the general 'script' memory to a particular occasion (see p. 21).

From the second year of life onwards, children's language and thinking abilities increase rapidly. This results in a major leap forwards in their memory capacities. They now can talk with others about their experiences. Initially this is usually their primary carer. In so doing, they organise and refresh their memories about events that they have experienced. Also, memories become more secure, organised and more accessible for reporting to others. It is likely, though, that events that are unspoken and remain secret will be less organised and structured in terms of memory and therefore more prone to be forgotten, or at least harder for the child to access and retrieve for later conversation.

Children's ability to retrieve memories from storage improves throughout the pre-school years and into early childhood. They learn strategies and methods that help them to recall personal experiences and events. Children become increasingly efficient at developing ways to encode information, store and rehearse it and then subsequently retrieve it, by such techniques as grouping things, linking information with other concepts or schemata, as it were in their own filing system, and by selecting certain central information for later recall.

A further area of particular relevance to practitioners is children's developing capacity to identify the source of a memory of an event or experience. For example, although an event or experience can be recalled, exactly when, where, with whom, or whether imagined, thought about or directly experienced, may be less clearly delineated in the developing child's mind. Adults still make source monitoring errors, but young children, especially pre-schoolers, are relatively more likely to be confused as to the exact source of their memories. This particularly happens when memories themselves are about similar events, if the memories in question are not strong, or if children are subject to powerful suggestion from adults around them. Source errors are more likely to occur too when recalling peripheral as opposed to the most personally salient aspects of an event. The ability to distinguish accurately the source of one's memory and then communicate this to another improves throughout the early years, so that by middle childhood most children have this ability. However, both adults and children can become confused over the source of their memories, especially in circumstances that increase suggestibility or foster confusion (Lindsay, 2002).

The impact of stress on children's memory has been the subject of much debate and contrasting findings, as well as views from different commentators. Overall, it appears that stress does not necessarily hinder memory and in some circumstances memories of stressful events are more vivid than memories of non-stressful ones. As the stress becomes more and more negative and personally threatening, it appears that children's memories become focused to a greater extent on what they thought and felt about the experience, rather than the details of the event itself. This may lead to some difficulties for practitioners assessing a child who has been victimised.

There are added factors to be considered. As we have already noted, long-term accurate memories are best preserved when there is opportunity for rehearsal and where there is an atmosphere of support and encouragement (often absent among children who have experienced traumatic events). In addition, negative traumatic events are often repeated, frequent occurrences and therefore may be recalled as schemas or scripts, as opposed to specific events. For these reasons, children's memories of personally experienced, traumatic events may be less organised or readily accessible to verbal recall in response to a practitioner's questions than other events. In contrast, distinctive, single traumatic episodes are likely to be well remembered by children.

## Summary

Overall, older children remember more and are more resistant to suggestion than younger ones. However, children from the age of two years can recall events that they experience, with rapidly increasing accuracy, especially more personally meaningful ones. By approximately the age of eight years, children's capacity to encode, store and retrieve information is on a par with that of adults. From then on their knowledge of the world continues to increase and some will learn ever more sophisticated strategies for retrieval, and hence will be able to recall and communicate their memories better than younger children.

Children's capacity to encode, store and retrieve information is affected by their circumstances. Thus, physical, psychological and

Jones, D. P. H. (2003) *Communicating with Vulnerable Children*. London: Gaskell.

social factors affect memory capacity. Such factors include children's motivation and their interest level or ability to attend to the task. Younger children have less-well-developed retrieval abilities than older ones. Overall, there is no single memory system, but instead a set of processes and systems that allow children to recall and communicate their personal experiences. In this sense children's memories are rich seams of information but also subject to decay and distortion if not treated with due respect. If a child has been subjected to maltreatment, this in itself can significantly affect his or her capacity to encode and register experiences, store them in memory, and later on recall and retrieve them when talking with an adult practitioner.

Memory capacity is significantly linked with language and communication ability. Nowhere is this more salient for practitioners than in the area of retrieval, where, even when a child is able to remember events, there may be significant difficulties in communicating them to an adult (see p. 22 ff.).

## Implications for practitioners

- Keep communication within the child's range of abilities.
- Always bear in mind the child's level of understanding and capacity to recall.
- Be alert to misunderstandings and miscommunications.
- Free recall is preferable to specific questioning because it is more likely to encourage the child to retrieve autobiographical and episodic memory accurately.
- The events and experiences that children find personally salient may differ from practitioners' appraisals. This can be a source for misunderstanding, which is best averted by regarding the child as the expert, while also inviting free recall from the child wherever possible.
- Children may not be able to discern accurately the origin of their memories of events. This potentially leads to confusion and misunderstanding, although children's free recall is likely to clarify such difficulties if they are present.
- Aim to discourage children's general memories for how things normally happen (their memory of a routine, script or pattern of usual events). This may be difficult if adverse events have happened repeatedly, but strive instead to find ways of drawing the child's attention to specific events or occurrences (see p. 21).
- In order to assess the child's memory for a particular event, the professional has to understand the events and circumstances throughout the period from initial encoding through to retrieval (taking into account age, context, personal characteristics and stress during all these times).

# Suggestibility

Suggestibility has been defined as 'the degree to which the encoding, storage, retrieval, and reporting of events can be influenced by a range of internal and external factors (Ceci & Bruck, 1995). A series of psychological experiments have demonstrated that when children are asked questions about events they have experienced or witnessed, the type of question affects the accuracy of their answer. For example, if the questions are focused, and particularly if they are leading or introduce new information or false suppositions, then the children in the studies could be misled about what had actually occurred. Adults are also susceptible to these misleading influences. There appear to be three possible mechanisms underlying these observations. First, the child's original memory becomes overwritten or destroyed by the new, suggested information, thus either supplanting it or creating a blended memory of both original and suggested information. Second, the original information may not have entered the child's memory in the first place and hence the suggested information is simply new. Third, the original and suggested information exist side by side in memory but when the child attempts to recall, it is the most recent, suggested information that is reported. It is probable that mixtures of all three occur in real life – new suggested information, original and accurate experience, as well as a blend of new and original.

---

**Box 2.2** Circumstances in which children are especially susceptible to suggestion

Children are susceptible to suggestion when:

- An adult repeatedly makes false suggestions (through misleading questions) and creates stereotypes about a person (Leichtman & Ceci, 1995).
- They are asked repeatedly to visualise fictitious events (Ceci et al, 1994).
- They are asked about personal events that happened a long time previously and their memory has not been 'refreshed' since (Bruck et al, 1995a).
- They are suggestively asked to use anatomically detailed dolls to re-enact an event (Bruck et al, 1995b).
- They are questioned by a biased interviewer who pursues a 'hypothesis' or line of questioning single-mindedly (White et al, 1997).
- They are questioned in an over-authoritative manner, or by an adult with perceived high status (Ceci & Bruck, 1995: pp. 152–159; Poole & Lamb, 1998, pp. 61–62).
- Their memories are not strong or recent.
- Practitioners communicate their own moral judgements to children, for example if they imply that particular individuals have 'done bad or wrong things', have been shown to affect the accuracy of pre-school children recalling an event.

---

Jones, D. P. H. (2003) *Communicating with Vulnerable Children*. London: Gaskell.

In addition, children have particular difficulty in distinguishing the source of information in their memories and therefore find it more difficult than adults to distinguish their own experience from someone else's suggested one, or their own imagined one. These difficulties are termed *source monitoring* ones, and are a feature of both adult and child memory abilities.

Other factors are important to the question of the suggestibility of children. Children are generally deferential to adults; this applies more to younger children and those with impairments than, for example, teenagers. In addition there is the effect of authority – children may feel that they must accept any implied knowledge that the practitioner conveys. The means by which such 'projection' occurs may be verbal and non-verbal. This is especially important among children who may be maltreated or seriously disadvantaged, whose alertness to the subtle clues and expectations of adults can in some circumstances be increased. These children's problems will be discussed further in Chapter 4.

The susceptibility to the effects of suggestion are summarised in Box 2.2, and apply particularly to younger children.

## Implications for practitioners

In order to promote the accuracy of children's accounts, while minimising suggestion, interviewers should:

- Use approaches and questions that invite free report.
- Remember that directive questions may be necessary to establish detail, but should be non-leading and paired with open-ended questions or invitations.
- Avoid leading questions.
- Not pressurise or use coercive techniques.
- Take care with the use of adult authority.
- Maintain neutrality, but not indifference.
- Manage any bias and presumptions held about the child's experiences, and strive to maintain an open mind.
- Maintain an awareness of the circumstances in which children are vulnerable to suggestion.

## The consistency of children's recall over time

It is quite common for children to communicate more than once, and often to more than one person, their recall of adverse events. Does repeating the information reduce the accuracy of what is recalled? If there are differences between one account and another, how concerned should we be that the child is being inaccurate? It has been shown that accounts by children and adults with genuine experiences do have inconsistencies within them. At the same time, simple repetition and repeated recall are beneficial to maintaining information in memory over time. This is of course provided that the events are freely recalled rather than influenced by suggestive questioning, leading questions or by an attempt to mould the experience within a predetermined script. We can think about the issue of consistency over time in three interrelated ways:

- The consistency of children's recall in response to repeated interviews.
- Consistency if questions are repeated within the same interview with the child.
- Children's accounts of events that were frequently repeated rather than single experiences.

## Consistency over repeated interviews

If children are questioned in an open-ended, non-leading way, their accounts in different interview sessions are likely to remain accurate. They may, however, introduce different details in the different interviews. Younger children in particular have limited skills in retrieving information from memory and therefore recall slightly different experiences at different times. The caveat for practitioners is that if the child offered new detail only in response to a focused or leading question, then the information may not be accurate.

## Repeated questions within the same interview session

Here the effects are a much greater cause for concern because children, especially younger children or those with learning disabilities, come to assume that their first attempt to recall an event may have been inaccurate and, in their wish to accede to the interviewer's perceived authority or merely age difference, provide an inaccurate, changed response to further questions on the same issue. There are ways of reducing these suggestive influences, for example by interviewers pretending to have forgotten the child's first answer, and generally by ensuring that their verbal and non-verbal communication to the child conveys that the child is the expert and has the knowledge, not themselves. Thus, they may seek clarification by asking questions such as: 'I think I know what you mean, but just help me understand that a bit better', or 'I just want to make sure I understand what you are saying ...'.

## Repeated events

Children who have been maltreated have often experienced repeated episodes of maltreatment. Equally, those children who have witnessed

Jones, D. P. H. (2003) *Communicating with Vulnerable Children*. London: Gaskell.

events such as domestic violence frequently have done so on more than one occasion. Hence, when communicating with practitioners there are particular issues about consistency because the child memorises many individual events, and indeed comes to recall some events as becoming part of the script and 'what usually happens'. We know that script knowledge is more susceptible to suggestive influence and inaccuracy, and this raises particular challenges for practitioners. Frequently this can be seen to be the basis for apparently inconsistent responses from children when questioned about events that recurred repeatedly. The practitioner can help, however, by working together with the child to identify an individual event and then seek the details about that particular time.

This may be achieved by choosing an event that has particular salience for the child, perhaps because it is the most recent, it was the first or it was one linked to a memorable event, such as Christmas or a birthday, a first day in school or a change of class or house. In this way the interviewer can help the child to keep focused upon the process of recall, rather than recognition of a regular script or routine memory of events. At the same time, practitioners can avoid those techniques that are more likely to produce inaccurate responses (again, since repeated events are generally considered to be more susceptible to the influence of suggestion than single ones). This means avoiding leading or focused questions wherever possible and ensuring that the interviewer's authority or implied knowledge or understanding about what might generally have happened is kept strictly under control and not conveyed to the child. A further practice point is to give the child plenty of time to focus on a particular event, rather than rapidly moving from one event to another.

## Implications for practitioners

- More than one session or interview may enable the child to describe further information.
- If the interview is of good quality, then no reduction in accuracy is likely to come from further interviews.
- If leading or suggestive techniques are used, then accuracy may decline sharply.
- Care is required when repeating questions about one issue during a single interview. If this is necessary, use methods that avoid suggestion or which may lead the child to assume a particular response is sought.
- Adverse events that occurred repeatedly present particular challenges for practitioners. Use techniques that allow the child to describe different aspects of their overall experience and assist them to distinguish memorable occasions.

- Take care with repeated questions, especially if questions require 'yes' or 'no' answers, or are in other ways focused or leading.
- Exercise care with questions that require the child to disagree (negative term insertion questions or tag questions – see below).
- Avoid questions that presuppose information.
- 'WH' questions (i.e. 'who', 'what', 'where', 'when') are generally satisfactory but exercise care with 'why' questions.

## Language development

Language issues are of great importance in this area of work. There are several useful extended discussions of salient language issues (Walker, 1994; Warren *et al*, 1996; Poole & Lamb, 1998, pp. 153–180; Walker & Hunt, 1998; Bourg *et al*, 1999). Here we will consider selected issues.

It is clear that, if interviewers speak in too complex a way, children, especially young children or those with learning difficulties, are likely to become confused. Poole & Lamb (1998) stress that it is not only complexity that is problematic, but also the usual way in which adults communicate with children. Everyday conversations with children are normally instructive or conducted on the basis that the adult knows the facts and the situation. Conversations are mainly designed to confirm that which the adult already knows. Adults normally use lots of specific questions and rarely invite children to be the 'expert'. However, when considering the possibility of maltreatment or trauma, the child is the expert and the adult genuinely does not know as much as the child, even though the child may think that he or she does. This is a critical difference and will be reflected in the linguistic style of successful interviewers.

Language comprehension and expressive ability develop rapidly over the first few years of life. The following are some landmarks. By the age of six years, the average child has a working vocabulary of around 14,000 words, having begun with spontaneous babble at around five or six months, spoken the first meaningful sounds or words at around one year, put three words together by around the age of two years, and constructed more complex sentences linking two or more simple ideas together by around the age of four. Children usually understand more words than they use (unless they have some specific problem with language comprehension). At the same time children may use a word differently from an adult. They sometimes include a broader range of meanings within their use of one word, or alternatively a much more restricted use. For example, a four- or five-year-old child may say 'no' when asked if an event occurred in his house because in fact the event in question happened in a flat, not a house. Throughout childhood, but especially in the pre-school years, children learn that language is more than mere words and grammatical rules. Language assists social relationships and rapidly helps the child develop further reasoning skills.

There is great variation between individuals, as with all aspects of development. A common difference between individuals is with respect to their general level of understanding and intelligence. It is well recognised that there is a link between a child's general level of intelligence and language ability. These differences are then manifested in terms of both speech and language and the child's general knowledge and reasoning ability. They are most marked in those children with learning impairments. Variation is accentuated further in those with speech and language problems, especially those with comprehension difficulties, who may appear more able than they truly are. Such children sometimes converse normally, belying significant difficulties in their capacity to understand adults.

Hence, it is desirable to know as much as possible about the child's language and communication ability before attempting an interview. Usually this will involve obtaining information from family members and the child's school or nursery before communicating with a child the practitioner does not know. Speech and language therapists may have especially valuable input, particularly for disabled children (this term is preferred to 'children with a disability' – see Chapter 5). Failing this, the practitioner can assess the child's level of ability through discussion of neutral subjects, such as a holiday or an event of interest that occurred recently, during the phase of initial assessment or during the introductory parts of interview sessions. Generally, however, it is difficult for practitioners to do all this within a single session; therefore it is preferable to have gathered information first from sources who have known the child longer.

Further variation is evident with those children whose first language is not the interviewer's. Aldridge & Wood (1998) provide discussion and advice for practitioners working with these children, as well as with those who are bilingual. Bilingual children often appear fully confident in the practitioner's choice of language, but this may disguise subtle difficulties in communication ability and level of understanding. Aldridge & Wood (1998) discuss these issues in the context of children who are bilingual in Welsh and English.

## Differences between adults and children

Notwithstanding the differences between individual children, there remain important differences between adult practitioners and children with respect to language. They are significant in the genesis of misunderstanding and the production of inaccurate or erroneous accounts from children. It is suggested here that if practitioners are aware of these differences, some potential misunderstandings can be averted. We can consider these differences under the following headings.

- Intelligibility.
- Grammar and vocabulary.
- Conversational style.
- Ability to detect and cope with misunderstanding.

## Intelligibility

The adult practitioner frequently does not understand the younger child's communications. This can be because a number of different areas of language are still developing. In the first place, the child may simply be unable to articulate particular sounds, for example the 'r' sound. Similarly, words that involve blended consonants are difficult for young children to pronounce and can lead to confusion; for example 'stop' may sound like 'top' or 'slam' may sound like 'lamb'. Children generally recognise different consonants and vowels before they can pronounce them themselves. This can create difficulties for practitioners if they repeat something that the child has said in an attempt to understand it better. Because children are still learning how to pronounce different words they may omit certain sounds from words, add new ones, substitute sounds, or mix them in order to convey meaning and communicate with adults. All of these processes can cause great difficulties for practitioners.

One three-year-old child was describing what had happened when a stranger had abducted her. She said she they had got sweets 'at golco'. Several weeks later it became clear from the subsequent police investigation that the suspect had stopped at a golf course, during the crime. This is a good example because the adult does not usually associate a golf course with a place where sweets might be bought. In this instance simply recording what the child said, without attempting to make further sense of it, allowed the account to be clarified over time.

## Grammar and vocabulary

The rules of grammar are gradually learnt during childhood. Vocabulary increases rapidly, especially in the years between three and ten. However, children and adults sometimes use the same word in order to mean different things. When children are learning how to use words they frequently use them before they understand their meaning. Pre-school children frequently omit the '-ed' from the end of a verb, before they have learned the use of past tense. Further, children have difficulty understanding the meaning of adults' words if they themselves have not yet incorporated them into their own vocabulary. Hence the choice of words by practitioners is especially important. Children may also use words as members of a list of words, such as the days of the week, without fully comprehending the concepts they signify.

## Conversational style

The conversational style between adults and children has already been mentioned. Adults normally talk with children in order to confirm their assumptions, often correcting children's communications as the conversation proceeds. When communicating with children about adverse experiences, as we have noted, it is the child who is the expert, not the adult, and so the rules are substantially different. Social practice enters the equation, too, so that children who do not understand the meaning of the practitioner's word may arbitrarily answer 'yes' or 'no' if they think they should, or that that is what the interviewer expects. For example, consider the children who, in one study, answered, in error, 'yes' to the question 'Did he touch your private parts?' In this experiment the interviewer had not touched the child's genital area. But when some children answered 'yes' they probably did so because they simply did not know the meaning of the phrase 'private parts' (Goodman *et al*, 1992).

## Ability to detect and cope with misunderstanding

Children also develop in their ability to notice, and manage, mis-understandings. Whereas adults will generally correct one another during conversations if one does not understand the other, children have less developed, and initially less effective, methods of coping with misunderstandings. Thus, instead of asking for clarification if they do not understand or merely saying they do not understand, they attempt to answer the question and may do so arbitrarily. They understand that it is the basic rule that it is their turn now to answer the question but have not yet developed the capacity to question or correct the adult. This effect is seen particularly when the adult uses complex language, or long sentences with embedded subclauses. It is also more likely to occur if the adult is of high authority in the eyes of the child. This last tendency can probably be modified to some extent through the professional conveying an attitude, throughout the interview, that it is the child who is the expert, not the practitioner. It is helpful to use phrases such as 'If I get something wrong, you tell me' or 'Sometimes I get muddled up, so you must tell me if I do'.

## *Communications that may lead to misunderstandings*

There are a number of words or types of conversation that have been found to be problematic in communications with children. They either cause misleading answers or are simply non-productive. This does not mean to say that use of these will always create problems, for they may be useful or appropriate in particular situations. It is merely that greater care may need to be taken with them, and interviewers should be aware of the limitations of using such language and the potential perils. The following is a summary of research findings in this area. For further discussion of these, see Walker (1994, pp. 21–50), Aldridge & Wood (1998, pp. 107–187), Poole & Lamb (1998, pp. 162–168) and Walker & Hunt (1998).

## Communications about touch

This is a key area for practitioners exploring the possibility of adverse events. Hence numerous difficulties have emerged when looking at communications between adults and children where the possibility of harmful touch and physical contact is being explored. Children below the age of six years may believe that it is only hands that can 'touch', and therefore exclude from their replies penetrative acts or touch by other parts of the body, or by implements. Equally, children do not necessarily have a well-developed idea about their internal anatomy and so they may, confusingly, say that a person put the penis or a hand 'inside' them, or 'in' them, when they mean between their legs or on them. Confusion may also arise because children may be quite literal concerning the direction of a particular action. For example, a younger child asked if she placed her mouth on the alleged offender's penis may answer 'no' simply because from her perspective it was the adult who placed his penis in her mouth (see Berliner & Barbieri, 1984). In addition, there may be legitimate reasons for touching the intimate areas of very young children or of children who are sick or disabled. These situations will require exploration with particular sensitivity.

## Communications about time

These may also cause difficulties for children under five years, who cannot necessarily understand past and future tense, far less concepts of frequency such as 'always' or 'sometimes'. Similarly, recounting order and sequence may prove difficult. Accurate responses to questions about time do not normally develop until the teenage years. However, even pre-school children can indirectly communicate about time by being asked to link their memories of events concretely to something else, such as whether it was dark or light outside, which house they were living in at the time, whether it was the holidays or school time, or what was on television, and so on. Young children tend to use the word 'yesterday' to mean anything that happened in the past before today, and 'tomorrow' to mean something that is going to happen in the future. However, they do recognise the word 'today' in the way in which adults do.

## Complex sentences

Simple sentences are better understood than complex ones. In particular, complex sentences that are long or contain 'tags' at the end or branches in their middle are especially complex and difficult for children to understand. One example would be 'He touched you there, did he?' – the tag at the end converts the question into a 'yes/no' one and also suggests the answer 'yes'. An example of a question with an embedded clause would be 'When daddy did that, and mummy was at work, where were you?'

## Ambiguous words

Some simple words can also present difficulties. For example, the word 'any' has been noted to be surprisingly complex for children, partly because such words are wide ranging and ask the child to search for every possibility. Additionally, this simple word may be used in a variety of ways by children and adults, so introducing particular levels of difficulty. Prepositions cause many problems, especially for younger children, who may use words such as 'above' and 'below', 'before' and 'after', in different ways from adult questioners. Part of the problem arises because pre-school children acquire the words before they have full understanding of the 'rules' for their usage.

## Comparisons

Words and questions that invite a comparison may prove difficult, especially with pre-school children. Poole & Lamb (1998) suggest using a multiple-choice question rather than an open-ended question if frequency or comparison is being sought. For example, 'Did that happen more than one time?' may be better phrased as 'Did that happen one time or more than one time?'

## Passive voice

Understanding of passive forms of verbs is not often well developed in younger children. It is generally observed that full command of the passive voice is not developed until teenage years (and in this author's case, and that of many adults, much later!). Interviewers should therefore use the active forms of verbs as far as they can in sentence structure. This has sometimes been called the 'noun/verb/noun' strategy. For example, 'Was she hurt by him?' would be better rephrased as 'Did John hurt her?'

## Asking about individual people

Children may have more than one person in mind when they use the word 'Daddy' or 'Mummy'. Practitioners will need to identify the person further through the use of another name, or by linking to time or place. Similarly, some people in the child's life will have more than one name. This can be confusing for the practitioner. Some of these areas of confusion are likely to be covered through prior discussion with the child's parent, carer or schoolteacher.

### 'Can you ...?' questions

Walker & Hunt (1998) have drawn attention to the use of 'Can you ... ?' They suggests these are substituted with 'Tell me about ...' type of questions because of the issue of expectations and authority which may be conveyed by using the phrase 'Can you ...?'

### 'Remember' questions

Requests for children to remember also present difficulties. It is thought that children do not use this word in the way that adults do until they are approximately nine years old (Walker, 1994).

### 'WH' questions ('who', 'what', 'where', 'when', 'how', 'why', 'how many', 'how much', 'whose')

'WH' questions are of particular interest because they are so frequently used by practitioners in interviews. Generally, 'what', 'who' and 'where' questions are understood by children first (by approximately three years of age), followed by 'when', and then 'how' and 'why' questions. The reason for this is probably because the latter types of question are associated with more complex ideas and relatively abstract concepts. 'When' questions have already been discussed (see Communications about time, above). 'Why' questions are difficult for many children and may be especially problematic for children who have been induced to feel guilty in the context of family violence, or perhaps to feel that the acts or events under discussion are in some way their own fault (see Chapter 4).

Asking children 'How many times ...?' can be problematic because they have to recall and reflect on past experiences and attempt to relay a number to the practitioner. It is probably preferable to ask whether something 'happened one time, or more than one time?', and then to steer the child towards one particular event (see Repeated events, p. 20).

## Implications for practitioners

- Misunderstanding in communication is common in both directions between adults and children.
- Misunderstandings in communication are not likely to be corrected by children, especially younger children.
- Adults need to simplify language and to check and continually monitor the child's understanding if they are unsure of the accuracy of the child's response.
- Practitioners should avoid abstract questions, hypothetical ones, complex comparisons across time and questions that involve taking another's perspective (unless the abilities are clearly within the child's capacity).

- Conversations, using the child's and the practitioner's own words, should be carefully documented, and the sequence preserved. True meaning may emerge only later on, when further facts are revealed.
- Avoid guessing or supposing what the child might have said. If unintelligible, simply ask the child to repeat the word/phrase and record it in order to clarify later.
- Use normal speech and avoid 'baby' talk.
- Children may pronounce words differently from adults. Therefore clarify words with possible second meanings through a follow-up question (e.g. 'Help me understand that a bit better' or 'Tell me more about that').
- Children and adults may use the same word differently. Children's usage may be more restrictive; for example, 'swimming suits', 'shoes', 'pyjamas' or 'night-clothes' may not be clothes to the child, and only 'hands' may be capable of touching. At the same time, other aspects of language usage may be more inclusive (e.g. 'in' might be 'between') or be simply special or idiosyncratic to the child.
- Avoid introducing new words for people, or objects, until the child has first used them.
- Certain types of words and concepts present difficulties for children below the age of eight to ten years, especially timing, words for comparisons, prepositions and words for touch, time and sequence.
- When children mention people, follow-up questions should be used to confirm their identity, such as 'Which daddy?' or 'Which house does the daddy who did that live in?' or 'Does that uncle have another name?'
- Active tense should be used rather than passive; for example, use 'When daddy hurt mummy' rather than 'When mummy was hurt by daddy'.
- Complex sentences that involve embedded clauses, multiple ideas, double negatives and 'tags' are especially problematic, for example 'Now when daddy, when he was drinking, and hurt mummy, did he not protect you from uncle Joe, even though uncle Joe was nice to you at other times?'
- Use 'WH' questions with care and ensure that the child can understand the complexity of the question; 'who', 'what' and 'where' questions are grasped earlier than are 'when', 'how' and 'why' questions. 'Why' questions may prove especially problematic for traumatised and abused children.
- Language and communication are about social relationships as well as the communication of understanding and memory. Hence, practitioners need to take account of the child's understanding of the social nature of the interchange, and avoid excessive authority or expectations of compliance.

- Cultural factors can be relevant and may need to be taken into account when considering the child's understanding of the rules of conversation.
- Avoid correcting or interrupting children, in order to encourage free recall and to convey the importance of the child's expertise rather than the practitioner's.

## Social and emotional development

The overall process of social and emotional development comprises the development of a close attachment to one or more carers in the first year of life, followed by the development of a secure sense of self up to the age of three years, peer relationships between three and seven, and the integration of these three between the ages of seven and 12 (Cicchetti, 1989). This is a very broad subject and we will highlight here only those issues that are relevant to communication with children in interviews.

Pre-schoolers are likely to experience more insecurity when separated from parents than older children. This will have an influence on whether, and in what way, young children are seen individually. Young children's capacity to trust an adult interviewer, and to feel safe enough to communicate, is also similarly less well developed than that of older children. This may mean that flexibility is required with children under five years regarding the number of interviews and the presence of parents as support persons.

Children under 10–11 years are more susceptible to social pressures, both because of a wish to please and comply with the perceived demands of adults around them and because of their reaction to adult authority. Hence, although support from the interviewer is helpful, it also renders younger children vulnerable to adult authority. This susceptibility is elevated when adult support is immediately combined with misleading questions or statements from the interviewer, or when the child is offered inducements to cooperate. The negative effects of these pressures can be attenuated through prior instruction, for example if the child is encouraged to correct the interviewer if he or she gets it wrong, or if the child does not agree with the interviewer's interpretation of events (Saywitz & Snyder, 1993; Saywitz, 1995). Nonetheless, there are clear indications for those communicating with children in these situations to use support carefully and to avoid linking it with any misleading suggestions.

Older children, particularly adolescents, have an increasingly sophisticated understanding of the consequences of their speaking with an interviewer about a sensitive or traumatic matter. Hence children who previously felt free to communicate are subject to different pressures in

Jones, D. P. H. (2003) *Communicating with Vulnerable Children*. London: Gaskell.

adolescence. These pressures may lead to inhibition of responses as young people weigh the consequences, to themselves and others, of disclosing information. This inhibition is enhanced by adolescents' greater reliance on same-age friendships for support and advice in challenging circumstances.

Children's handling of perceived *secrets* mirrors some of these developments (for a review see Bussey, 1992). For example, young children may not appreciate the need to keep a secret, unless required to do so by a carer, in which case their loyalty is impressive (Ceci & Bruck, 1995). In experimental situations, where children between the ages of three and six years were asked to keep secrets, the younger children were not consistently affected by this, nor by whether they were subsequently interviewed in a leading way. However, children around five or six years did withhold more information when a parent told them to do so. However, they too were not particularly affected by suggestive or leading questions (Bottoms *et al*, 2002). Whether these results could be generalised to situations involving possible victim-isation of a child is open to question.

As children's knowledge of the world increases, moral development becomes more universal and less oriented towards the parent figure. As reliance on a single carer for security lessens, the child of middle school years becomes less likely to obey parental admonitions to keep secrets. However, as teenage years approach other considerations come into the picture, in particular the more refined reflections of the teenager who contemplates the consequences of accusing someone, or disclosing a secret, in relation to the moral imperative to speak the truth. Children under the age of six years may, therefore, reveal secrets quite readily, unless they are required to keep them by a parent figure to whom they are attached. Children between six and 12 are less driven by loyalty to a carer, but by teenage years will be affected by considerations about the social consequences of revealing a secret that now makes the moral choice more difficult for them.

## Conclusions

Practitioners' competence and confidence are greatly enhanced by an understanding of children's development. Although perhaps initially daunting, the implementation of an appreciation of developmental factors and differences results in communications with children that are both more fruitful and safer from errors.

Not every professional will possess skills in communicating with children in all different phases of development. It is therefore important to know one's limitations and to have the confidence and ability to access those with the requisite skills when this is necessary.

An overview of the kind given here can obscure the considerable individual differences between children. This is one of the reasons why knowledge of one's own children, grandchildren or those of friends is simply insufficient and can lead to misleading generalisations. A broad base of experience and knowledge is necessary and this may have training implications, as well as implications for those planning services. It may be important to consider how practitioners can gain experience if it has not been a core part of their training to date. One way may be through structured observation of young children and pre-school children in nursery class or child development centres. Similarly, much can be gained from multidisciplinary discussion and the obtaining of both start-up and continuing training (Davies *et al*, 1998).

# CHAPTER 3

# Erroneous concerns and cases

Errors do occur in processes of assessment and decision making about whether a child has been maltreated. False or erroneous concerns and conclusions about maltreatment are important, both for the harm that they cause and because if they can be better understood there is a chance to prevent their occurrence. Both false negative and false positive errors occur, and each has the potential to result in substantial harm for the child and any adults involved. In the case of false negatives this includes the continuation of abuse. False positives can result in unnecessary separation of child and parents, as well as parental or carer loss of job, reputation and important relationships, and possibly even imprisonment. Although it has been stated that a number of false positives is the price to be paid for an effective child protection system, it is surely the case that the objectives must be to reduce false positives to an absolute minimum, to seek better ways of identifying genuine cases, and to identify false positives as rapidly as possible. Complacency about the existence of false positives severely undermines public and professional confidence in child welfare and protection processes. Interestingly, the extent of psychological harm deriving from false positives has not been systematically studied, although it is likely to be considerable. In what follows, the focus is on false positives, or erroneous conclusions that a child has been abused.

We first look at the terminology used in this area and the consequences of erroneous concern. We then briefly review the frequency with which these kinds of errors seem to occur, before considering what is known about the mechanisms or processes leading to erroneous conclusions. This chapter ends with a summary of implications for practitioners.

## Terminology

The language that has been used to describe false negative and false positive judgements of maltreatment has been both varied and in many instances pejorative. For example, a deliberate wish to deceive is implied by the term 'false allegation'. Motivation in these instances is complex and, where possible to establish, ranges from deliberate lying and a wish to deceive through to mistaken assumptions, including those deriving from faulty professional processes. Normally, false positive judgements have been called 'false' or 'fictitious allegations or accounts', although sometimes the term 'unsubstantiated allegation' or similar terms have been used. We have preferred the term 'erroneous concern' or 'erroneous case of maltreatment' because these are neutral and invite appropriate questions as to motivation or mechanisms leading to error, rather than inferring deliberate or malicious falsification (Oates *et al*, 2000; Westcott & Jones, 2003).

## The consequences of erroneous concern

There are several stages that follow a referral for possible maltreatment to a professional agency, up to that agency's eventual conclusion as to whether concern is justified. Errors leading to false positive conclusions can occur at any point in this process. In principle, erroneous concern is not necessarily harmful for either child or adult, depending on how it is assessed and managed. However, if an adult loses a job or is off work for an extended period, or loses a foster care licence, or if a child is unnecessarily placed in substitute care, then erroneous concern can be seen to have seriously detrimental effects. As a referral progresses from initial concern to a final conclusion about whether it constitutes a case of actual abuse, then it is likely that any negative consequences of an error will increase. In fact, we know that many concerns are determined to be erroneous at a relatively early stage in the process and without negative consequences for child or adult (Jones & McGraw, 1987; Oates *et al*, 2000).

The task, then, is to identify insubstantial or erroneous concerns early in their journey through the professional system, before secondary harm occurs. This implies keeping major state actions (e.g. reception into care, arrest of suspects) in abeyance for as long as possible, relative to child safety imperatives, while the nature of the initial concern is being fully assessed. This is probably feasible, providing practitioners are aware of the possibility of error and avoid reaching premature conclusions.

## Frequency of types of false positive errors

The outcomes of assessments and investigations of suspected maltreatment are normally classified in terms of whether they are substantiated or not (Ceci & Friedman, 2000). In the field of child sexual abuse, approximately 40% of all concerns will be substantiated by an agency after investigation (Ceci & Friedman, 2000). Rates of substantiation by child welfare agencies show some variation between countries, and over the past decade. However, in general, between a third and a half of the concerns about possible maltreatment that are presented to child welfare agencies become substantiated after assessment.

Oates *et al* (2000), in a study of 551 instances of concern about possible sexual abuse that were presented to one child protection agency in the USA, found that 43% of concerns were substantiated. The remainder represented a variety of situations which, although previously designated under the all-inclusive umbrella of 'unsubstantiated', could be classified so as to distinguish: erroneous concerns emanating from children; cases where abuse was thought definitely not or very unlikely to have occurred, which these authors termed 'not substantiated'; and, finally, the inconclusive cases. Errors emanating from children constituted 2.5% of all referrals. Thirty-four per cent of cases were 'not substantiated'; these were a mixed group and included concerns made in good faith but which, nonetheless, on assessment had been made in error, through to mistakes by the professional system and finally deliberate lies or distorted concerns in relation to referrals by adults. The data did not allow for a more detailed analysis of this mixed group of not substantiated cases. Finally, there was a group, 21% of all referrals, where there was insufficient clinical evidence to place the concern in any one of the other categories – and these were the inconclusive cases.

Overall, studies have found that the rate of substantiation is higher for referrals about possible sexual/physical abuse, yet lower for suspected neglect and, in particular, emotional abuse.

It is possible to distinguish four broad categories of concern:

- *Substantiated concerns*. Those that, after assessment, are held to be cases of child abuse or neglect.
- *Erroneous concerns by children*. These arise from a child's mistaken concern, or by children in conjunction with their parent(s) or carer. These also include deliberate lies or attempts at deception made by children.
- *Erroneous concerns by adults*. In these situations child maltreatment is considered to have definitely not, or probably not, occurred, because of error by either the referrer or the professional who evaluated the concern. Referrers' errors range from concerns made in good faith, through mistaken assumptions to deliberate deceptions, malicious referrals and lies. Professional errors are of judgement and response, including but not limited to problems in interviewing techniques.
- *Inconclusive concerns*. These are situations were there is uncertainty or insufficient clinical evidence to place the referred concern into any one of the above three categories.

Oates *et al* (2000) contended that classifying the outcome of referrals in ways such as those above would assist practitioners to detect errors earlier and thereby lessen the potentially harmful side-effects of assessing and intervening. Further studies are necessary in order to confirm this proposition.

# Mechanisms leading to false positive cases of abuse

There are a variety of mechanisms that have been described as contributing to both erroneous concerns and cases of maltreatment. This is a difficult area to study, not least because there is no absolute test of accuracy, or criterion of truthfulness, only degrees of certainty that a case might be genuine or fictitious/erroneous (Jones & McGraw, 1987). However, some studies have tried to overcome these obstacles (Jones & McGraw, 1987; Oates *et al*, 2000; Hershkowitz, 2001). It is from studies such as these that the causes or mechanisms listed in the previous section have been derived. More than one mechanism may contribute to a single false positive cases (e.g., Hershkowitz, 2001). Table 3.1 sets out the mechanisms that have been described.

Mistaken concerns can develop from the child, the parent or carer, or from a professional (e.g. if a child starts behaving out of character). They may also emerge from difficulties in relationships or in interaction between child and adult, perhaps because of language or communication difficulties. It can be helpful to distinguish erroneous or false accounts from mere assents by children that give rise to a false conclusion by an adult (Pezdek & Hinz, 2002).

Children do lie. Vrij (2002) has reviewed the research on children's abilities to be deceptive. Vrij notes that children are capable of being deliberately deceptive by approximately the age of four years, but do so rather simplistically, and without the capacity to convince others that they are not lying until they are older. It has been suggested that there are at least five different reasons for children to lie (see Vrij, 2002):

**Table 3.1** Mechanisms through which erroneous cases occur

| Source of error | Mechanism |
| --- | --- |
| Deriving from child | Lying<br>Mistaken assumptions (sometimes in conjunction with carer)<br>Source attribution errors (see p. 15)<br>Erroneous assents |
| Deriving from parent/carer | Lying<br>Mistaken assumptions (uncomplicated mistakes; biased perspectives; delusional states) |
| Deriving from professional | Mistaken assumptions<br>Incompetence (bias, leading and suggestive questions and techniques, inadequate investigation) |

Jones, D. P. H. (2003) *Communicating with Vulnerable Children*. London: Gaskell.

- To avoid negative consequences (e.g. punishment).
- To obtain a reward.
- To protect their self-esteem.
- To maintain relationships (e.g. 'white lies').
- To conform to norms and conventions.

Younger children tend to lie to avoid punishment, and children progress through the list above so that it is not until secondary school that children tell lies to maintain norms and conventions. Even very young children will lie to protect people whom they love (Ceci & DeSimone Leichtman, 1992).

In some cases more than one mechanism can be seen to have contributed to the false positive.

## Implications for practitioners

- Erroneous or false accounts about maltreatment do occur.
- They occur because of mistaken concerns, beliefs, assumptions or conclusions, as well as because a child or adult (or both) lies.
- Erroneous concerns from adults appear to be more common than those emanating from children.
- Knowledge about the reasons why children deliberately lie can alert practitioners to the potential for lies to occur.
- The potentially harmful consequences from erroneous concerns can be minimised through high-quality assessments and investigations.
- Neutrality and managing presumption and bias within assessments or investigations are the key requirements to prevent harmful outcomes from concerns made in error.
- Practitioners should develop processes for preventing initial concerns becoming translated into erroneous conclusions or cases (false cases) of abuse.
- Errors may be false positive concerns or conclusions or false negative ones. Positive errors can have significant effects on both child and adult, while false negatives are likely to lead to continuing harm to the child.
- Expanding the range of possible conclusions for assessments, from substantiated or not, to include other gradations may help practitioners detect errors at an earlier stage.
- Practitioners can help prevent errors through high-quality communications with children, and through processes that are designed to reduce bias and presumption.

# CHAPTER 4

# The child's psychological condition

The child's psychological condition can affect communication in a number of ways. Children who are exposed to adversity can be psychologically affected by it. These effects, in turn, have an impact on children's capacity to communicate, as well as the professional's capacity to understand and respond to them. As we shall see, children respond very variably to specific kinds of victimisation, or exposure to adversity, and hence it is not possible to generalise about psychological effects on the child. Nonetheless, there are differences among children who have been exposed to different forms of adversity that distinguish them from their peers and that are seen with varying degrees of frequency.

Some of the effects on children result in psychological conditions or social behaviours that render children more difficult to communicate with, or to listen and respond to, for example children who, as a consequence of maltreatment and other adversity, have significant behavioural or conduct problems or difficulties resulting from drug use, or who frequently resort to lying or deception. Besides these effects of adversity and direct victimisation on children, there are children who have coexisting psychological or psychiatric disorders, who present significant challenges for the professional. Examples include hyperactive or emotionally disturbed children. Finally, there are children who are reluctant communicators or who are simply un-communicative, for a variety of reasons.

First in this chapter, the effects on children of different forms of adversity are considered, to the extent that they may be relevant to professionals seeking to communicate with them.

## The effects of adverse experiences on children

Although a wide range of negative adverse events occur to children, we are mainly concerned here with those that involve victimisation of the child. 'Victimisation' has been defined as 'harms that occur to individuals because of other human actors behaving in a way that violate social norms' (Finkelhor & Kendall-Tackett, 1997). The key points are that victimisation is caused or created by other humans and that it involves some form of social deviation. In this sense these kind of adverse events are different from other traumas and losses such as illness, death, natural disasters and accidents. A range of motivations may lie behind the human actions against the child, but these frequently involve issues of moral judgement, legality and social justice. Not surprisingly, therefore, the consequences cross a number of boundaries between agencies, disciplines and social institutions (Finkelhor & Kendall-Tackett, 1997; Hamby & Finkelhor, 2000). While there has been a substantial increase in interest in the general field of victimisation (for an introductory summary see Mezey & Robbins, 2000), there has been rather less consideration of the impact of victimisation from a developmental perspective throughout the life span.

Finkelhor & Kendall-Tackett (1997) have sought to organise the general way of thinking about the impact of victimisation according to its effect in four different dimensions of a child's life. This can be a useful way of thinking about victimisation and its impact on children, which takes one beyond the mere listing of symptoms and psychological problems. The proposed four dimensions are as follows:

- *Appraisals* of the victimisation. Children at different developmental levels understand and appraise their experience of victimisation differently, for example with respect to how morally wrong, or otherwise, they feel the activity was and the extent to which they feel a sense of self-blame.
- The *impact of victimisation on the child's current developmental status*. Children at different stages of development are involved with different fundamental tasks: pre-school children with attachment to a carer, three- to six-year-old children with self-recognition and development, and older children with peer relationships. Victimisation at different points is known to affect children differently.
- *Coping strategies*. Children at different phases of development have different repertoires available to them with which to respond to stress. Additionally, there is good evidence for major individual differences in coping strategies between children of the same age.
- *Environmental factors*. These include the immediate family and wider social context surrounding children when they are victimised and the way in which these affect the child's responses.

Finkelhor & Kendall-Tackett proposed this framework in order to emphasise the aspects of victimisation most affected by developmental processes, rather than to offer a fully comprehensive model. For example, the severity, duration and frequency of victimisation experiences are likely to have substantial effects on outcome, too. Nonetheless, the approach is presented here so that the scope and impact of victimisation experiences on children may be appreciated more fully. A key factor when considering victimisation is that one type of harm rarely occurs in isolation, either at the time of its occurrence or in terms of subsequent events. It is known, for example, that there is substantial crossover between different forms of child maltreatment and between child maltreatment itself and other forms of family violence, such as domestic violence and even elder abuse. Equally, a longitudinal study of the impact of child maltreatment on the developing young person into adult life has emphasised that effects vary substantially according to whether subsequent life events add to the primary trauma or ameliorate its impact on the child (Fergusson & Mullen, 1999).

Notwithstanding these difficulties, victimisation experiences do affect how children subsequently appraise and think about the events that occurred. They can affect the child's ability to negotiate important developmental stages (Cicchetti & Toth, 1995). They affect the child's coping strategies (perhaps leading to dissociation: Putnam, 1997; Macfie *et al*, 2001) and lead to symptoms of psychological distress, as well as affecting cognitive function and personality development. Table 4.1 sets out the psychological impairments and problems that have been associated with childhood abuse.

**Table 4.1** Psychological impairments and problems associated with childhood abuse

|  | Childhood impairment | Adult impairment |
| --- | --- | --- |
| Affective symptoms | Fears<br>PTSD<br>Depression | Anxiety<br>PTSD<br>Depression |
| Behaviour problems | Conduct disorder<br>Sexualised behaviour<br>Self-destructiveness<br>Hyperactivity | Aggressive conduct<br>Self-destructiveness<br>Alcohol/substance misuse |
| Cognitive functioning | Educational problems<br>Language difficulties | Educational underachievement |
| Personality and social adjustment | Self-esteem<br>Attachment<br>Peer relations | Pregnancy before 19 years of age<br>Sexual aggression<br>Prostitution<br>Parenting problems<br>Somatisation<br>Personality disorder<br>Revictimisation<br>Sexual problems |

From Jones, D. P. H. (2000b) Child abuse and neglect. In M. Gelder, J. Lopez-Ibor & N. Andreasen (eds), *The New Oxford Textbook of Psychiatry* (pp. 1825–1834). Oxford: Oxford University Press.
PTSD, post-traumatic stress disorder

---

**Box 4.1** Possible effects of domestic violence upon children

- Increased symptoms of anxiety, post-traumatic stress disorder (PTSD).
- Conduct and behaviour problems.
- Hyperactivity (though this has been less firmly established).
- Educational problems – aggressiveness, concentration and attention problems, school non-attendance.
- Problems controlling and regulating emotion (particularly anger, but also fearfulness).
- Self-blame and low self-esteem.

---

Some of the effects of domestic violence on children are set out in Box 4.1.

Naturally many of the effects listed in Box 4.1 are compounded by a range of other problems facing families in which domestic violence occurs (Jouriles *et al*, 2001).

The overall implication from these studies is that children who are victimised may be significantly affected in their development, adjustment and psychological functioning. While this may be demonstrated in terms of symptoms of behavioural or emotional difficulty, there may also be substantial effects on the way the young child perceives events, reacts to problems and has learnt to cope with stresses. All these have implications for practitioners. These are listed below, according to the child's phase of development.

## *Implications for practitioners*

### Children aged under three years

Although many practitioners will not be seeing children under the age of three, if this phase of development is disrupted by victimisation experiences, problems with attachment are likely to persist into later childhood and so the effects listed below will remain salient.

- Child abuse, neglect and family violence can all affect children's ability to form a normal attachment to their parents or carers. They may become excessively clingy and unable to leave the carer's side, or simply not attached to any adult figure and possibly indiscriminate in their affections.
- Behaviour difficulties such as excessive aggression and tantrums with prolonged episodes of loss of control.
- Emotional symptoms such as excessive fearfulness and nighttime waking.

### Three- to seven-year-old children

Problems in the areas below affect communication ability and present challenges for practitioners. While these problems can be caused by other factors besides victimisation, they are more common among victimised children.

- Behaviour difficulties, such as aggression and oppositionalism.
- Emotional problems, such as excessive fearfulness, nighttime disturbance, persistent anxiety and sometimes post-traumatic stress symptoms.
- Poor self-esteem.
- Dissociation.
- Poor adjustment at nursery and pre-school.

### Children aged seven years and above

Difficulties such as these can create major problems for communication and assessments. Children may be excessively and apparently idiosyncratically affected by practitioners' approaches. Special care is needed with physical reassurance and touch, which may well be misinterpreted by a child who has been maltreated. Touch is in fact best avoided. Older children are likely to be excessively mistrustful.

- Behaviour problems, such as aggressiveness and oppositionalism.
- Emotional difficulties, such as anxiety, excessive fearfulness, post-traumatic stress reactions and sleep problems.
- Depression and pervasive feelings of worthlessness and helplessness.
- Self-blame, leading on to self-harm.
- Lack of trust in relationships.
- Indiscriminate friendships and relationships.
- Unpopularity and isolation from peer group and difficulty sustaining friendships.

## Some special problems

Special problems occur when children have been threatened, coerced, manipulated or bribed to maintain loyalties or to keep secrets.

Children who have become dissociated in response to long-standing maltreatment prove difficult to interview and may experience major problems concentrating and attending to task, and recalling past events. Some show unusual or unexpected emotional reactions to those events that are recalled, perhaps appearing bland or unusually calm.

Children with severe symptoms of post-traumatic stress disorder (PTSD) can find the recall process traumatic in itself and seek to avoid painful and disturbing memories at all costs.

Children who have come to blame themselves for the victimisation they have experienced can be hard to communicate with, as they may feel substantial guilt and self-reproach in association with memories of victimisation. A small minority of children may have harmed others (sexually, physically or emotionally), either as part of their own abuse or because of subsequent behaviour difficulties. For such children the experience of victimisation is accompanied by its perpetration. Such children are especially difficult to communicate with.

Older children may have found schools, police or other agencies unhelpful or even negative in the past. This may affect their willingness and capacity to communicate during the current assessment.

# The effect of the child's psychological condition on communication

The child's psychological condition can have a major effect on the success of attempts to communicate. Mental health difficulties are common in childhood: they affect up to 20% of children and young people in urban areas, although lesser rates are found in non-deprived social settings. While victimisation, trauma and adverse experiences are more common in children with mental health difficulties, they are but one of a variety of factors that can cause them. Maltreated children and those who live in particularly adverse circumstances are more likely to suffer from conduct and behaviour problems, or from excessive fearfulness or PTSD, or to show symptoms of attention deficit hyperactivity disorder (ADHD). However, some of these conditions may have causes other than trauma and adversity.

For other children, the experience of adversity is less clearly linked to the fact that they have a psychological condition or mental health problem. Autism is one example. Regardless of the cause, children's mental health problems can present difficulties for practitioners assessing them. In the section that follows we consider different symptom groups, or types of presentation, together with implications for practitioners and the strategies that may be useful in meeting these challenges.

## Children with behaviour problems

Behaviour problems are frequently demonstrated through excessive aggressiveness, hostility or oppositional behaviour. In older children these behaviours can be accompanied by substance misuse.

### Implications for practitioners

- Most children with significant behaviour problems will need no special arrangements for assessment over and above ordinary good practice, because the behaviour disturbance is likely to be situational.

- Sometimes, the presence of a support person for the child or young person is useful and occasionally necessary to protect the interviewer (either because of the child's level of aggression or because of the possibility of allegations of abuse by the child).
- Children with behaviour problems may benefit from greater care being taken in the explanation of the rationale for their assessment.
- Practitioners should seek to involve the child or young person as far as possible in decisions about where and how an assessment should take place. The aim is to achieve as much of a sense of mutual partnership as possible.
- The gender of the practitioner should always be considered as to whether there are any special implications for the child.
- With severely behaviourally disturbed children, the practitioner should avoid overt confrontation, but be gently firm concerning boundaries as to what is acceptable or permissible behaviour within the assessment session.
- Some children are attention seeking and distractible. The best approach is to ignore everything that is attention seeking and at the same time respond positively and with interest to positive and appropriate behaviour from the child.

## Hyperactive children

The activity level of children can be increased for a number of reasons, including anxiety and fearfulness, or as part of general behaviour difficulties. The activity level is often raised among children with a learning disability. Children with ADHD are constantly restless, unable to attend to one task and are sometimes impulsive, too.

### Implications for practitioners

- Remember that although the intelligence level of hyperactive children is generally normal, some may have accompanying problems with their language and level of understanding.
- Aim to achieve a calm, focused session in which the child can appreciate and understand its purpose.
- It is preferable not to spend too long on unfocused periods or unstructured breaks, which may encourage hyperactive behaviour.
- Avoid having too many distractions in the assessment session. Remove extraneous objects and allow access to only one toy or drawing at a time.
- The support of a person whose presence is known to help the child to focus can be useful. This may be one of the child's

relatives but could quite possibly be a teacher or other supportive adult. However, the disadvantages of a support person should also be considered, for example the potential for distortion, disruption or constraint on what the child communicates.

- Consider whether to seek the help of a professional who is experienced in managing disturbed and hyperactive children.
- You should keep the sessions relatively short and have frequent breaks. It may be best to plan to divide preparation and rapport building from any definitive assessment interview.
- Some children with ADHD have accompanying behaviour difficulties. For these children the suggestions made above for interviewing children with behaviour problems may help in addition.
- Choose moments to slow the pace of the interview, by focusing and helping to draw the child's attention to one specific incident or time that the child has just mentioned. This should be done sparingly, however, because children with ADHD have little or no ability to control their level of attention. Hence, if you continually require the child to slow down, the child will not be able to achieve this and further agitation and distress can result.
- Maintaining eye contact can be an important way of helping the hyperactive child to focus.

## Emotionally disturbed children

Children can become emotionally disturbed in a wide variety of ways, especially if they have been victimised. Common problems are excessive anxiety and tearfulness, PTSD, dissociation and depressed states of mind. Some apparently anxious children are also hyperactive and so the methods described above may assist these anxious children, too.

Some children suffering from fearfulness or anxiety are difficult to form a rapport with. Children with PTSD or dissociation may suddenly develop excessive fears at particular times during the assessment, perhaps when recalling adverse events. Depressed young people may have difficulty seeing any point to communication and rapport with such children can be hard to establish. Also, helpless negativity may pervade the assessment. Occasionally thoughts and intentions of self-harm are expressed.

### Implications for practitioners

- It is preferable to know as much as possible about the child's psychological condition before any assessment is made. Has there been any recent change? The more information interviewers have, the better they can understand the child's condition and respond sensitively to it (see Chapter 11).

- It is best to be gentle, yet clear about the purpose and focus of the assessment.
- Sensitivity to the effect of eye contact is necessary. It may be difficult for emotionally disturbed children to tolerate direct eye gaze with the interviewer. The use of drawings or other tasks can helpfully divert and move the centre of attention from between interviewer and child to a more neutral third space. Sometimes communication while walking or driving a car achieves the same purpose. Overall, it may be necessary to avoid appearing over-intrusive or overbearing, and at the same time to give the child more space than normal.
- It will be necessary to go at the child's pace, not the interviewer's, as well as to respect the child's right to remain silent. Although these points apply to all children, they become more salient with emotionally troubled children.
- If the child seems to show excessive distress when communicating about particular topics, the practitioner should respect this. The interviewer may be able to return to sensitive topics again, if and when the child is ready to do so.
- It is preferable to close an interview successfully rather than end one in disarray. Even if the interviewer's hopes and agenda were not achieved, it is preferable to close the interview well and possibly return after a break or on another day.
- The rapport-gaining phase of an assessment interview may take longer with severely emotionally disturbed children than with those who are not so disturbed.
- Some children develop particular responses to individual professionals of a type that can render an assessment impossible. For example, some children with severe anxiety symptoms or post-traumatic stress reactions may have powerful and overwhelming responses to individual interviewers, perhaps because of their gender or one of their individual characteristics. While effective rapport building can sometimes overcome these difficulties, it may be necessary to reconsider who is the best professional to undertake the assessment, and to change the arrangements if necessary.

## Reluctant or uncommunicative children

Children may be reluctant to engage or participate in an assessment for many reasons. Some such children will have significant emotional difficulties and the approaches suggested in the sections above may well be applicable. Others may have been encouraged, coerced or even bribed not to communicate, or perhaps have always lived in a culture where to cooperate with 'the welfare', or other agents of the state's authority, is derided or fundamentally discouraged. Some children are not so much reluctant to communicate, but in fact have nothing to say – that is, the concern about the child and the situation has arisen in error (Chapter 3).

The central issue for the practitioner is to contemplate a broad variety of possible reasons why the child may be apparently un-communicative and reluctant to engage in the assessment. While this may seem self-evident, there have been many cases and situations described in both research (Ceci & Bruck, 1995) and in the world of practice (Jones & McGraw, 1987; Clyde, 1992; Ceci & Bruck, 1995) where erroneous conclusions of maltreatment have followed on from mistaken assumptions made by those who first assessed the child. Interviewer bias can easily affect the subsequent actions and can lead to the pursuit of the interviewer's agenda at the expense of the child's expressed reluctance.

## Implications for practitioners

- Attempt to understand why the child might be reluctant, or apparently uncommunicative. Consider a wide range of alternative or competing possibilities, including that the concerns giving rise to the need for assessment are unfounded or erroneous.
- Plan for additional time for gaining rapport. Several rapport-gaining sessions may be necessary in order to establish trust. More than one interview session may be necessary during an assessment. If this occurs, it is important to avoid excessive repeated questioning (see Chapter 3).
- Try to deal with impediments or obstacles. These include the child's concerns about confidentiality and the consequences of talking about particular adversities. The obstacle may be more general, in the form of an impoverished ability to trust others, or to believe the answers that you give to key questions. It can be helpful to involve the child as much as possible in the process of assessment. In this way, children whose experience of adults to date is one of exploitation may be able to communicate if they regain some control of and influence in the interview. Care should be taken not to promise more than can be delivered. Such approaches can be useful during an extended rapport-gaining phase.
- Sometimes explaining that you cannot help the child unless you can understand him/her better, or appreciate what difficulties he/she has, can be a useful approach. Again, care will be necessary to keep such explanations at a general level and not to introduce suggestive material.
- Maintaining a non-judgemental approach is essential. The child may take time to be assured that the interviewer has the ability to deal with difficult or sensitive material. This quality may need to

be demonstrated by the practitioner through responses to issues that are offered by the child. There can, in these circumstances, be a period of testing to see if the practitioner is 'up to the job'.

- Sometimes it is necessary to be persistent, although without hectoring the child.

- Know as much as possible about the child and family situation in advance. This enables the practitioner to anticipate many potential problems. For example, a child may have had previously negative experiences with professional assessments.

- The practitioner's own communications are important, both verbal and non-verbal. Professionals are frequently aware of the things they say but not of the more subtle messages they convey through facial expression, relative attentiveness, gesture and body movements. It can be instructive for practitioners to try to imagine how children see them.

- It is also useful for practitioners to understand their own reactions to difficult situations and types of responses from children. Often these echo personal experiences, resolved or otherwise. Professional supervision and peer support combined with personal understanding are especially important aspects of successful practice when dealing with challenging or reluctant children.

Jones, D. P. H. (2003) *Communicating with Vulnerable Children*. London: Gaskell.

# CHAPTER 5

# Diversity and difference: implications for practice

Britain is socially and culturally diverse, in many different respects, such as social class, race, cultural group, language, disability, and sensory ability. This should be taken account of when working with children and families (Department of Health, 1989; Department of Health *et al*, 1999, paras 7.24–7.26; Department of Health *et al*, 2000, paras 1.42, 1.43, 2.26–2.30, 2.31). Difference may result in children and their families being the subject of discrimination and, for some, this may be compounded as a result of their particular circumstances; for example, black disabled children may experience discrimination because of their race *and* because they are disabled (Department of Health *et al*, 2000, ch. 3).

Difference should be addressed by professionals at an early stage in order to ensure that the child is worked with in a respectful manner. In this chapter certain areas of diversity are selected in order to highlight the practice implications for those seeking to communicate with potentially victimised children. The reader is referred to specialist resources and to government guidance, research summaries and practice recommendations focusing on particular areas. Diversity and difference arising from race, culture and language are considered first, and then the challenges presented in work with disabled children who may have been victimised. It is important to stress at the outset, however, that not all black children or all those with sensory impairments, say, have difficulty in communicating their distress. Equally, not all practitioners find difficulty communicating with children in social or cultural groups different from their own. However, to the extent that difference does present a challenge, the reasons for it and some suggestions to help the practitioner either to prevent or to address discriminatory practice are set out here.

## Race, culture and language

'All children belong to a race. All children have a culture. These are important facts in the establishment of the identity of all children. However, in this country race and culture are discussed almost exclusively in relation to black

Jones, D. P. H. (2003) *Communicating with Vulnerable Children*. London: Gaskell.

**49**

and minority ethnic children. Why is this? The answer is simple. In this country 'whiteness' and English culture are seen as the norm. They represent the benchmark against which other communities are measured. If you are the 'norm' you do not have to think about your 'normality' because it is not you, but those who are different from you that are made conscious of their difference.' (Phillips, 1993)

It is clear that the cultural background of the participants is a key aspect of the context within which interviewer and interviewee communicate.

'Those from similar cultures can understand whether they are more readily and more likely to be attuned to the subtle nuances which guide social encounters. Likewise, the wider the disparity of cultural identity, the less common ground there will be, and hence the greater the potential for communication breakdown.' (Hargie & Tourish, 1999)

Curiously, there has been relatively little research on interviews with children from different racial or cultural groups from the practitioner. Commentators agree that different cultural conventions are likely to have an influence on the interaction between interviewer and interviewee, but there has been surprisingly little systematic research on how this might affect the outcome, or what processes might alleviate difficulties in communication. Even without such studies, it would clearly be a matter of good practice to raise awareness of racial and cultural issues among interviewers and to take appropriate steps to challenge discriminatory attitudes in practitioners and their organisations. However, a general exhortation is insufficient. It has been pointed out that there is a direct link between racism and those deficits in professional practice that are considered to have contributed to the deaths of some black children in recent enquiry reports (Dutt & Phillips, 2000). Dutt & Phillips address two key issues for practitioners in relation to black children and their families. First, what are the needs of black children and their families, and in what ways are these similar to, and different from, those of white children and their families? Second, how can these needs be accounted for when white practitioners work with black children and their families?

Before proceeding further, it is appropriate briefly to consider the range of terms and concepts that have been used when considering issues of race and culture.

- *Race* itself is a term that has been used to categorise humans by their physical characteristics and especially their skin colour. Aside from facial appearance and skin colour, though, there is little evidence for major biological differences between racial groupings. There is also a surprising lack of agreement on what characteristics define racial grouping.

- *Black* is used in the political sense to refer to all people of African and South Asian descent (Banks, 1999). However, others use the term to refer only to those with African/Caribbean origins.
- *Dual heritage* denotes those children with parents from more than one ethnic group. 'Mixed parentage' is also used. Dual heritage is commonly used to refer to black children who have one parent who is white and one who is black.
- *White* refers to people of white European descent.
- *Racial identity* describes the acquisition of an integrated sense of self in relation to race. Identity is a broad concept that in itself incorporates several related dimensions: racial, ethnic, cultural, religious and linguistic identity. *Individual identity* is linked with *group identification*, which describes the process by which individuals categorise one another, an element of which may be by race, culture or ethnicity (Dutt & Phillips, 2000).
- *Ethnicity* describes the group sense of coherence and 'belongingness' of persons who have a common geographical, historical and political background and interests.
- *Culture* refers to the rites, traditions, values, beliefs and customs that are shared by a group of people. It is important to note that not every person in a cultural group adopts the same values and beliefs, however. It is considered that cultural identity operates at both a group and an individual level (Dutt & Phillips, 2000). It is also important to recognise that culture evolves and changes over time (Banks, 1999).
- *Racism* is prejudice that is based on race. It is characterised by attitudes and beliefs about the inferior nature of persons of other races, although it may be restricted to fear of persons from different cultures. It can be helpful to think of individual, institutional and cultural racism. *Individual* racism refers to the irrational beliefs and discriminatory behaviour of a particular individual. *Institutional* racism refers to the existence of policies that discriminate or restrict the opportunities of an ethnic group. *Cultural* racism refers to the individual and institutional expression of superiority of one ethnic group over another. However, the key issue is in the effects and social consequences of racism, which generate prejudice and discrimination (Banks, 1999).

From the above it can be seen that the primary issues surround minority groupings and the relationships that exist between them and the majority cultural, ethnic or racial group. Hence, although the focus in recent times has been on black minority ethnic groups, many of the comments that follow can be applied or considered in relation to white minority ethnic groups. However, there are particular issues for black people in relation to racism in Britain and the significant impairment of life opportunities that has resulted from institutional racism (Macpherson, 1999). Hence while the emphasis is on minority black ethnic groups, reference is also made to other issues that emerge from difference. In fact, the lessons practitioners are able to draw from a better understanding of the racial and cultural issues affecting the black minority in Britain at present are likely to be of benefit for all minority groups.

'Issues of race and culture cannot be added to a list for separate consideration during an assessment, they are integral to the assessment itself. From referral through to core assessment, intervention and planning, race and culture have to be accounted for using a holistic frame for assessment. It is only through an active approach to the inclusion of race, culture, and identity in assessments that accuracy and balance in assessments of families can be achieved.' (Dutt & Phillips, 2000)

Farmer & Owen (1995) also underline the inappropriateness of adding issues of culture, race and ethnicity to a long list of items that need to be considered in assessment, and instead stress that they should be integrated into the whole perspective of every child and family.

There is evidence that black children experience more economic hardship than do the white majority. The black minority overall has more families on lower incomes, more unemployment, poorer housing and are more likely to be the victims of crime. They are also more likely to experience racism and bullying. Refugee children have higher rates of PTSD associated with past experiences before arriving in the UK. Notwithstanding these increased rates of disadvantage and of adverse experiences, there is some evidence that black children are less likely to be identified as victimised or abused. For example, rates of sexual abuse in epidemiologically sound surveys show little variation by ethnic or racial group. Nonetheless, in one UK-based study, black children were under-represented in referrals for suspected sexual abuse (Gibbons *et al*, 1995; Jones & Ramchandani, 1999).

For many ethnic minority children, issues of race and racism are further compounded by language differences (Aldridge & Wood, 1998). Linguistic issues may exist at a subtle level (Poole & Lamb, 1998, p. 176) and lead to difficulties in understanding between interviewer and child, or more overt difficulties where English is not the first language of the child but is the language of the interviewer. Poole & Lamb (1998) describe some examples of misunderstandings developing between white teachers and Hispanic-American children in relation to the meaning of direct gaze, seen as disrespectful in Hispanic culture, whereas white teachers considered the averted gaze as a sign of disrespect. The opportunities for misunderstanding and miscommunication can be even greater among bilingual children, especially those whose first language is not that the interviewer uses (Aldridge & Wood, 1998). Aldridge & Wood make the point that interviews are difficult enough for monolingual English-speaking children and their monolingual English-speaking interviewers, without the additional demands of being interviewed in a second language. It has also been suggested that bilingual children may benefit from being interviewed by someone who has bilingual ability too, so that the child is able to interchange language (a common characteristic of bilingual children). Moreover, if the child was victimised in the context of one language, possibly the 'home' language, it may be important for the child to describe it in that same language. This raises the issue of the use of interpreters, which may be important to consider, even for bilingual children. As in the area of disability, careful planning and communication between interpreter and interviewer are crucial.

## Implications for practitioners

- The overriding implication for practitioners from the foregoing is that appreciation of race, culture and language ought to be a natural quality permeating all aspects of professional practice and the agency in which practitioners operate. Knowing when additional, specialised help is required and how to access it locally is a key issue for individuals and their organisations.

- It is important that organisations and professional groups are not caught unawares by individual cases that suddenly bring issues of ethnicity, culture, religion or class difference into sharp relief. It is preferable for the group to have already developed awareness of ethnic and cultural variations in their client or service group, and of any differences from their own identity. In this way, individual issues emerge against a background of an informed professional culture, which does not then require a major shift of understanding or practice in order to appreciate the individual child or family.

- The consequence of an awareness of race and culture on the part of the professional should reduce down to a deep respect for the individual and their particular experiences, attitudes and expressed wishes and feelings, rather than aggregating individuals and assuming common qualities. Some children exposed to relentless pressure within their particular culture may find it easier to communicate with someone whom they perceive to be from a different culture. Equally, it will be important to determine which aspects of culture or racial difference are most salient for the individual. For example, an appreciation of religious faith may be especially important to some children, and be even more salient than race and racism per se.

- Organisationally, assessment services should seek to have male and female interviewers from the different cultural backgrounds present in their area. For less numerous minority groups there should be a clear line of access to the relevant expertise in terms of both cultural knowledge and linguistic expertise.

- Professionals sometimes avoid raising issues of race and culture because they feel uncomfortable themselves or because they think it might inhibit communication (Banks, 1999; Abney, 2002). In fact, the opposite is likely to be the outcome. Relief and gains in terms of rapport and trust often follow raising such issues with teenagers.

- It will be important to determine the extent to which the child has been exposed to racism. A black child who has experienced racism could find it extremely difficult to talk with a white interviewer. The experience of racism may have a major effect on trust and the development of rapport within the interview. A child's preferences should be taken into account. Stereotypical assumptions should not be made, however, because of the variety of experience within an identified racial or cultural group. Assuming that a black child must have experienced racism, and is therefore likely to have particular fears about white interviewers, would be tantamount to racism itself.

- There may be benefit in arranging for a combination of black and white professionals to have contact with a child and his or her family. This arrangement has the benefit of highlighting ethnic and cultural difference, while at the same time modelling a means for approaching and managing it.

- When undertaking assessments, information is necessary on the cultural, religious and language issues, and particular arrangements may have to be made to collect this. For bilingual children careful consideration will have to be given to which language should be used for an interview in each case.

- Family history and information about a child's cultural heritage are vital to an understanding of both personal and group identification. Dutt & Phillips (2000) emphasise the importance of understanding children's relationships within their social context, how much information children have about their own heritage, and the family structure in which they live, including links with other attachment figures and the impact of migration, separation and trauma, including illness and war, on children and their wider family network.

- Within an interview it may be important to ensure that any drawings or dolls present imagery from a variety of cultures and not just the predominant white culture. This point has also been made in relation to disabled children (Kennedy, 1992b).

- Initial assessments allow these issues to be explored in further detail and, most importantly with older children and teenagers, for the child's wishes and feelings to be determined.

# Disabled children

Children who have impairments that affect their communication may present difficulties for practitioners (Marchant & Jones, 2000). There are several interconnected reasons for this. The primary one, of course, is that such children can be more difficult to communicate with, for the practitioner, than other children. Accounts from disabled children who have poor communication skills can seem less convincing, or believable, than those of their non-impaired peers. Notwithstanding these challenges for practitioners, children with some degree of impairment or disability are more vulnerable to victimisation (Westcott & Jones, 1999).

This section is orientated to generalist practitioners, who should recognise that specialist consultative or direct help may well be required for individual children. Specialist resources are referred to throughout this chapter. Training packs are available that provide useful introductions to this area of work (ABCD Consortium, 1993; NSPCC/ Chailey Heritage, 1998; JRF, Triangle, & NSPCC, 2001).

The term 'disabled children' covers a wide range of impairments. It includes those with learning disabilities, and sensory and communication impairments, as well as those with physical disability. These impairments vary in the degree to which they affect communication ability, although all such children potentially suffer from the prejudices and biases of non-impaired adults who seek to communicate with them. Some disabled children can communicate well. This section first considers approaches to describing and conceptualising disability, before considering children with sensory impairment and those with learning disability. Implications for practitioners are summarised at the end.

## *The social model of disability*

The social model of disability is a useful framework for conceptualising and orientating oneself to the issues faced by disabled children (Westcott & Jones, 1999). In this perspective, social factors such as prejudice and discrimination are seen as key factors that define the child's identity and his/her perspective on the world. Prejudice and discrimination result in inequitable and inadequate access to a range of facilities, services and opportunities, such as employment, once children enter adulthood.

One consequence of adopting this social model is to use the term 'disabled children' in preference to 'children with disabilities'. This is because the impairment *is* an integral part of the child's identity, rather than something added on to an otherwise whole identity as a child.

Adopting a social model of disability permits the disabled child to be understood as a whole individual within the context of the family and culture. This has a major effect on professionals' views of the unique position of the particular child, taking into account the disability but also issues of sexuality and gender, race, culture, language and religion (see 'Recognising identity' in ABCD Consortium, 1993). Such a perspective enables the practitioner better to understand a child for whom more than one factor may lead to prejudice and loss of opportunity. For example, consider an Asian child who is also disabled (ABCD Consortium, 1993).

## World Health Organization's classification

The social model contrasts, but is not wholly at variance with, classification systems that are rooted in physical and medical approaches to disability. The World Health Organization's system (World Health Organization, 1980) conceptualises ill health at four levels: pathology, impairment, disability and handicap. While it is acknowledged that this represents a conceptual framework with areas of overlap, the definition of each of the four levels is as follows. *Pathology* refers to internal damage or disease within the person. *Impairment* refers to the physiological consequences of disease or disorder, leading to specific symptoms and signs. *Disability* is defined as 'any restriction or lack (resulting from an impairment) of ability to perform an activity within the range considered normal for a human being'. It also refers to the sense of distress and personal nuisance caused by the underlying condition. *Handicap* refers to the social consequences, and effects on social adjustment, of a particular disease or disorder (for a review and discussion see Wade, 1998).

The social model has a different perspective but tends to span disability and handicap in its conceptualisation of the meaning of 'disability'. The word 'impairment' is a focus of concern and debate among advocacy groups in the field of disability, because in part the notion of impairment conveys a derogatory meaning, and because of the difficulty in viewing a person's impairment separately from its social and political consequences. If used with awareness and as a way of objectively considering what biological functions might be different for the individual child and produce challenges for the interviewer, then it can be helpful.

## Importance of disability for practitioners

Disabled children are at greater risk than non-disabled children of maltreatment (Westcott & Jones, 1999). Furthermore, as noted, many practitioners experience greater difficulties when communicating with disabled children, especially those who do not have experience of working with such children and young people. Notwithstanding these difficulties, there is no reason to presume that the principles of good practice guiding communication with disabled children should be any different from those for non-disabled. Similarly, the progression of enquiry described in Chapters 9–11 should be the same. If that is so, what then is different?

In this brief chapter it is not possible to cover all the impairments or disabilities that affect children. Indeed, it may be inappropriate to stress impairment type at the expense of the options available for communication (JRF, Triangle & NSPCC, 2001). So here we will consider some of the issues relevant to children with sensory impairment by way of illustration, before returning to implications for the practitioner when communicating with disabled children with all varieties of impairment.

## Children with sensory impairment

Children with sensory impairments include those visually impaired, those hearing-impaired and those with multi-sensory impairment, that is, both deaf and blind. Sensory impairments have significant effects on children's development, especially those with the more profound degrees of impairment and those with sensory loss occurring in the early years of life. Sensory impaired children may have other associated conditions, such as learning disability and cerebral palsy, but not necessarily so. Children with multi-sensory impairment are more likely to have accompanying disabilities. Sensory impaired children are, therefore, a diverse group and it would be incorrect to make generalisations about their ability levels or capacity to communicate (Hindley & Brown, 1994). Nonetheless, language delays and variations are common. Visually impaired children are more likely to use standardised statements, to repeat words and phrases of the interviewer (echolalia) and reverse personal pronouns. Setting aside, for a moment, the reasons for these differences from non-impaired children, they are noted here in order to underline the challenges involved for practitioners when assessing children with these disabilities, and to emphasise the need for specialist skills.

Hearing-impaired children also show delays in language development. Even without formal sign language they are more likely to rely on visual spatial systems of communication. Within deaf communities across the Western world these have developed into specific sign languages. However, it must be remembered that British Sign Language (BSL), in common with other sign languages, is structurally different from spoken English. The languages also differ from one another. The individual hearing-impaired child will vary with respect to the extent to which sign language is the predominant or merely the shared means of communication with spoken language. This is because of the variation in educational practice, social experience and family environment of deaf children.

It has been pointed out (Kennedy, 1992a) that for work with hearing-impaired children to be effective, the following must be in place: a qualified interpreter (registered with the Council for the Advancement of Communication with Deaf People, CACDP); a social worker with deaf people to work cooperatively with the interviewer; full planning of interview questions with the interpreter; and more time for the interpreter with the child to determine the child's level of language development and preferred means of communication. Lastly, it is suggested that visual means of communication be used as much as possible (Kennedy, 1992a).

Hearing-impaired children may well have difficulty understanding abstract concepts, as a consequence of language delay (Kennedy, 1992a,b). As in other forms of sensory disability, hearing-impaired children appear to be exposed to less rich discussion and mutually rewarding conversation, particularly if they have mainly communicated with non-native signers. Hence, the performance of victimised children with a sensory disability may be significantly below their true ability to communicate their experiences, if those children had developed effective means of communication over time. Hence difficulties in communication between child and practitioner presenting at the point of initial assesment to explore whether a child has been harmed or not may have their roots in a lengthy history of impaired opportunities for development in communication extending back before any recent concerns emerged. One significant implication of this is that children with a sensory disability require more time, more effective interview planning and more extended introductory phases to any interviews. It is unlikely that work of this complexity can be conducted in a short space of time, or indeed in single sessions.

As with children with other kinds of disabilities, if accurate and complete accounts of adverse experiences are sought it is preferable to plan for several sessions, in addition to the time required to evaluate the child's ability and to establish trust, as opposed to condensing professional efforts into a single session. The proviso, however, is that extending the process of assessment in this way places a greater premium on preparing both child and family, and providing continuing support and advice, in order to minimise the likelihood of any suggestion (see Chapter 2) or undue influence on the child's memory of events between sessions.

Comparison studies have indicated that hearing-impaired children can provide accurate and complete accounts of traumatic events (Porter *et al*, 1995). However, the accuracy of the hearing-impaired children was reduced as the questions became more focused and directive. This may have been because the children had a greater desire to please or engage the interviewer or because they were more creative and imaginative in their responses. Alternatively, the inherent suggestiveness of the method of communication, in this case American Sign Language, could have influenced the outcome. This emphasises the need for careful planning and the involvement of interpreters before starting work with such children. In this way, the least suggestive methods are used. In addition, pairing direct questions with open-ended invitations is equally relevant among disabled children as it is among non-disabled children.

## Augmentative communications systems

A variety of systems of communication other than sign language and speech are used with some disabled children. Augmentative communication includes any system or tool that either supplements or replaces traditional communication methods. Frequently, now, these involve alphabet and symbol communication aids which are either in the form of boards or, increasingly, computerised. A variety of such communication systems exist. There is also great variation in the extent to which these communication systems are closer to spoken language in terms of grammar and syntax, or closer to sign language. Once again, this emphasises the importance of having the assistance of a qualified interpreter as well as a practitioner familiar with the particular impairment the child has or method of communication used. It is also suggested that practitioners have additional training in the particular area of disability involved. It has been pointed out that many of these communication systems do not include sufficient vocabulary on sexual or abuse-related matters, which can be a limitation for assessments about adversity or possible victimisation (Kennedy, 1992a,b; Marchant & Page, 1992). There have been attempts to adapt existing systems in order to respond to these concerns.

It will be necessary to assess whether the child has sufficient cognitive ability to respond to questions about possible maltreatment. This may not be immediately clear if the augmentative communication system does not contain a sufficient range of language to enable the child to convey victimisation experiences (however, with careful planning and the use of a skilled interpreter it is usually possible to make a decision about this). A second difficulty is determining the extent to which communication can occur using augmentative communication free from suggestive influence (Poole & Lamb, 1998). If doubt exists about this, a second opinion from an independent specialist, knowledgeable in both the area of disability and the communication system in question, should be sought (Poole & Lamb, 1998). This particular issue has been a major one for those working with children displaying autism (Jones, 1994), where a technique

Jones, D. P. H. (2003) *Communicating with Vulnerable Children*. London: Gaskell.

**59**

known as facilitated communication has been in vogue (see special issue of *Child Abuse and Neglect*, 1994, issue number 6, on this topic).

## Other types of and aids to communication

On occasion, interviewers find that they cannot communicate effectively with some disabled children. While professionals strive to find alternative methods of effective communication, we remain reliant on indirect methods of assessment for some children. These children will, therefore, not be able to be involved in investigative interviews conducted for criminal justice purposes (Home Office *et al*, 2002), but should nonetheless be worked with using more indirect methods of assessment, which will sometimes inform decisions about their safety (see, for example, Kennedy, 1992a,b; Howlin & Clements, 1994).

The cognitive interview is a structured interviewing technique designed to increase the quantity and quality of information that adults and children recall. It relies on methods that improve retrieval techniques from memory and, therefore, should theoretically be of assistance to those with learning disabilities. At present the technique is not available for use by all practitioners in the field, although several of its methods have found their way into other schemes of interviewing (Memon, 1998; Poole & Lamb, 1998; Milne, 1999). Additionally, the cognitive interview begins with introductory techniques that are designed to protect children from the effects of misleading questions. It has proved effective in experimental studies with children with mild learning disabilities (Milne & Bull, 1996; Price, 1997, cited in Milne, 1999), and so this technique may prove useful in the future, once further field studies have been conducted.

## Implications for practitioners

Interviewers communicating with disabled children require an awareness of the total situation of the disabled child, including experiences, attitudes and expectations of helping professionals. However, the individual child may or may not have typical experiences and expectations. This understanding should not lead to a new set of stereotypical views or pre-judgements about disabled children – albeit those informed by disability or awareness groups. Box 5.1 summarises issues that may present difficult challenges for interviewers when working with disabled children.

The principles guiding good practice for in-depth interviews, and the approach to enquiry set out in Chapters 9–12, should hold good for disabled children, as much as for non-impaired children. It is their *application* that may need to be adapted. There is little research to guide practitioners and to help them decide what adaptations are necessary.

> **Box 5.1** Consequences of a child's impairment that present challenges for practitioners
>
> - Practitioners' lack of familiarity with disabilities can lead them to feel ill at ease and deskilled. This in turn can affect their own and the child's capacity for successful communication.
> - Practitioners' low expectations, stereotypical views and assumptions about disabled children's abilities sometimes result in communication difficulties.
> - Lack of appreciation of the disabled child's identity and how this might affect the child's views and expectations of the world can affect the child's performance.
> - Among children who are interviewed by professionals (and where, unusually, the child is the expert, not the adult), the disabled child is likely to be less familiar than non-impaired children with practitioners who seem to want to know about their views and experiences. This can affect all aspects of interviewing, but particularly establishing an initial rapport and the ground rules for initial assessments.
> - The disabled child's expectations of adults (e.g. expectations that adults are likely to misjudge abilities; make unwarranted assumptions, based on stereotypical ideas; or that they are likely to be patronising) may reduce the child's willingness to communicate or overcome barriers to trust.
> - Disabled children are at greater risk of abuse by carers than are non-disabled children. The experience of abuse will reduce their responsiveness and trust in authority and helping professionals. Rapport and ease of communication are thus affected.
> - The disabled child may have difficulty communicating per se, notwithstanding help and support available.
> - The child's psychological condition is sometimes perceived to be a consequence or an inevitable correlate of their disability, rather than a sequel of maltreatment (ABCD Consortium, 1993, pp. 66, 83–87; Howlin & Clements, 1994).
> - Disabled children are more likely to be compliant with adult expectations (as they are perceived by the child) due to dependency for core needs and expectations for compliance in personal and intimate care, and education.
> - The disabled child's dependency, combined with isolation and lack of knowledge of alternatives, leads to fear of loss and reluctance to disclose adverse experiences (Kennedy, in ABCD Consortium, 1993, p. 28).

Some of these involve changes at the strategic planning level, while others refer to the detail of the practitioner's communication with a disabled child.

Principles that guide good practice are set out in Boxes 5.2 and 5.3, based on the best evidence available for communicating with disabled children. However, for these approaches to be effective they must be put into practice in the context of a cultural change within child welfare agencies, and the gap between child protection professionals and disability-focused professionals must be bridged (Marchant & Page, 1997; Milne,

1999; Department of Health, 2000). These approaches must also be supported by an effective training programme (ABCD Consortium, 1993). The items listed in Boxes 5.2 and 5.3 have been drawn from the few reviews of this particular area (Marchant & Page, 1997; Poole & Lamb, 1998, pp. 199–202; Milne, 1999; Westcott & Jones, 1999).

---

**Box 5.2** Good practice at the organisational planning level

- Ensure the availability of interview settings for disabled children that can cater for their individual needs (e.g. a ground-floor suite, doors sufficiently wide for wheelchair access, appropriate toileting and personal care facilities).
- Ensure that arrangements are in place for specialist help to be available for front-line workers, either for consultation or for direct work.
- Plan for longer periods of time, and for more visits, than might be set aside for interviewing non-impaired children.
- It can be helpful to have either (or preferably both) selected practitioners trained to communicate with children who have particular impairments, or access to specialists in the child's specific condition or form of communication, who can act as observers, consultants, communicators or interpreter (Kennedy, 1993).
- Setting up exchange arrangements with neighbouring assessment teams can lead to a wider 'bank' of appropriately trained practitioners with experience of particular impairments.
- At the same time, awareness by all members of a practice team of the issues involved for disabled children is important, so that the assessment of disabled children's concerns does not become marginalised or solely deflected on to selected individuals.

---

Jones, D. P. H. (2003) *Communicating with Vulnerable Children*. London: Gaskell.

**Box 5.3** Good practice for individual practitioners

- When planning assessment sessions with disabled children, major efforts are required in order to obtain an understanding of the meaning that disability has for the individual child, as well as specific information on the nature and degree of the impairment.
- Check that the facilities are adapted to the child's needs.
- Check the arrangements for selecting the best time of day, food and drink, as well as personal care needs.
- Ensure that there is a preparatory stage, in order to provide time to liaise fully with the relevant specialist to advise the interviewer how to modify communication for the individual child.
- Arrange for the possibility that more time than usual may be required for gaining rapport.
- Similarly, a longer period may be required for establishing the ground rules and reiterating them during the session.
- Three ground rules are especially important in work with disabled children: that it is perfectly acceptable both to say 'I don't know' and to seek clarification, and agreeing simple means to communicate the need for a break.
- Place especial emphasis on establishing a relaxed atmosphere, without pressurising influences (Milne & Bull, 1996; Poole & Lamb, 1998).
- It is appropriate to have more reliance on collateral information to assess the likelihood of any maltreatment (Howlin & Clements, 1994; Westcott & Jones, 1999).
- Indirect assessments of the possibility of maltreatment may be required in order to augment direct assessment interviewing (for example, assessing susceptibility to suggestion during a standardised cognitive test – see Howlin & Jones, 1996).
- With children with a learning disability, especial care must be taken over their acquiescence to and compliance with the interviewer, especially in relation to 'yes/no' questions (Bull, 1995). (These children tend to choose the last of any two options. Hence vary the order in direct questions. The 'either/or' question format is preferable to those which invite a 'yes/no' answer.)
- Pictorial 'either/or' formats may be more fruitful than verbal presentation of choices.
- Use short sentences and preferably not compound ones.
- Take care with personal pronouns – use full names instead (i.e. first and surname, or other means to clarify identities).
- Mark topic changes explicitly, for example using phrases such as 'I want to ask you about something else now'.
- Children with learning disabilities are more vulnerable to suggestive questions. Hence, use open-ended prompts and encouragement, with questions such as 'Is there a way to tell me more?', 'Is there a way to show what you mean?' or 'Perhaps you can show me what you mean?'

Jones, D. P. H. (2003) *Communicating with Vulnerable Children*. London: Gaskell.

**63**

# Successful communication: core skills and basic principles

There is a great deal known and a remarkable degree of consensus about the core skills and central features of high-quality communications with children. For instance, Angold (1994) summarised best practice thus: 'The art of good clinical interviewing lies in the ability to combine the efficient collection of reported information, an observant eye and the projection of interest and concern about the child's problems'.

Direct communication with children is part of many professionals' work. Teachers, psychologists, psychiatrists, nurses, children's guardians, social workers and others all communicate with children individually as one part of their work. Each service has built on the core skills described in this chapter to develop particular methods and techniques that are salient to the profession's particular purpose. Although the work of teachers, child psychologists, social workers and children's guardians is clearly distinct, there are, at the centre of their direct work with children, similar qualities and skills that can be identified as core.

These consist of a mixture of individual skills and personal qualities. The emphasis in this book is on assessments and communications with children where there is a possibility of victimisation or other adverse experiences. The quality of early communications is vitally important for a number of interrelated reasons. First, they are important from the child's perspective, especially if the child has harboured a secret or distressing information for a period of time before mustering sufficient courage or developing enough trust to communicate their concerns (Department of Health, 1995; Sharland et al, 1996; Wade & Westcott, 1997). Second, the success of the initial communication will act as a foundation for future intervention, with respect to the child's and the immediate carer's capacity to trust the professional system subsequently (Sharland et al, 1996). Third, when children have been victimised through sexual abuse, and sometimes physical or psychological abuse, they are the main witnesses and there are unlikely to be other sources of information readily forthcoming. Hence, the child's account is of critical importance (Jones, 1992) and will only occasionally be corroborated.

Jones, D. P. H. (2003) *Communicating with Vulnerable Children*. London: Gaskell.

**Box 6.1** Core skills and qualities professionals need to communicate effectively with children

- Listening to the child.
- Conveying genuine interest.
- Empathic concern.
- Understanding.
- Emotional warmth.
- Respect for the child.
- Capacity to manage and contain the assessment.
- Awareness of the entire transaction between interviewer and child.
- Self-management.
- Technique.

Fourth, once a child's account has been distorted by poor communication it is very difficult, if not impossible, to retrieve the original memory of events (Ceci & Friedman, 2000). Fifth, there are significant sequelae that are dependent upon the child's account, such as decisions concerning contact and residence with loved ones for the children, and the possible pursuit of criminal proceedings, combined with jeopardy to employment, for the adults. Hence, the quality of the original communication is of very great importance.

Communicating with children can be viewed as one example of an interpersonal skill. In this sense interviewing children is similar to any other skilled performance to the extent that it involves the following qualities: fluency, rapidity, automaticity, simultaneity and knowledge.

The core skills and qualities are listed in Box 6.1. These qualities overlap, to varying degrees. It is also proposed here that the skills and qualities possessed by the professional are interdependent. The professional will require all the skills and qualities considered below in order to communicate effectively with children.

The *capacity to listen* is central. Listening is a quality that pervades all the others discussed below. Effective listening involves a combination of timing, interest, attending to the child and being prepared to absorb what is communicated. It also involves a readiness to wait for the child to speak and to tolerate silent periods, as well as the ability to avoid making interruptions, or at least to restrain them. Listening provides the child with time to respond, without being hastened by the practitioner. It usually includes care and modulation of speech, so that the child is not overwhelmed or inhibited. Children who have sensitive or traumatic experiences to impart can be highly attuned to the professional's ability to listen effectively. Effective listening is underpinned by openness, open-mindedness and an absence of bias (see paragraph on self-management, below).

The Cleveland enquiry report pointed to the need for interviewers of children to have an aptitude for this work (Butler-Sloss, 1988). One aspect of this quality is a *genuine interest* and curiosity in the individual child and his/her world. It is probably a prerequisite for effective communication with children. The interest has to be genuine and not contrived, for children will soon recognise feigned interest. Interest may be cultivated, and impediments to its genuine development revealed through supervision and peer review, and thereby is potentially modifiable.

*Empathy* is the ability to identify with and understand the child's thoughts and feelings. It is thought to involve both understanding and an emotional sensitivity on the part of the professional. It also incorporates the ability to convey these qualities to the child.

Conveying *understanding* is important. The child will need to feel that 'something important about him or her has been understood by someone who cares and is willing, and perhaps able, to help' (Angold, 1994). This is a complex series of intertwined qualities and capacities but includes the fact that the interviewer comprehends the child's communications, has sufficient knowledge about the subject being communicated and has the technical ability to gather the data efficiently. Developmental awareness is obviously key to understanding. The professional also needs to appreciate the overall context within which the interaction between the child and the professional is occurring (Cox, 1994). Understanding involves combining these bases of knowledge and skill with the previous three qualities.

*Emotional warmth* is a necessary component. It does not have to be excessive, and probably ought not to be, especially if a child has been abused within a context of charm and seduction. It has been found that too much warmth causes discomfort for some and may cause them to stop talking or expressing feelings. A balance is therefore required between excessive warmth and cold indifference (Cox, 1994; Shemmings, 1998). This balance is likely to be different for each child and will require sensitive attunement on the adult's part.

*Respect* for the individual child's personal differences is a necessary ingredient. This may involve sensitivity to a child's cultural or communication difference or an impairment. It also may involve addressing the child's need for understanding or for particular timing in relation to the progress of the assessment. One avenue for bringing this into relief is through discussion about consent, particularly with older children and adolescents.

The capacity to *manage the assessment* is important so as to allay and contain the child's anxieties or concerns. It is closely linked with the capacity to organise the session in a way that the child can engage with and feel a necessary degree of comfort.

Jones, D. P. H. (2003) *Communicating with Vulnerable Children*. London: Gaskell.

It is important for professionals to develop their *personal awareness of the entire transaction* between themselves and the child. Hargie & Tourish (1999) have emphasised that practitioners have actively to develop their skills as interviewers if they are to maintain and expand their awareness of the transaction. The perceptive skills required include the capacity for self-monitoring, the ability to evaluate others in an objective way, and a third quality that they term 'meta-perception'. For the last skill the professional is able to look down on the entire interaction between the child and professional and understand the reciprocal perception process: how the child might be perceiving the practitioner and what the child seems to think about the adult's perception of him/her.

Self-management and technique will be discussed under seperate headings, as they require more detailed discussion. Self-management is an essential quality for professionals to acquire and continue to develop when working with children who have suffered adversity.

# Self-management

*Self-management* includes both the capacity for self-monitoring and the managing of personal emotions, thoughts, attitudes, values and belief systems, especially those that might interfere with the particular interview task in hand. Being aware of and managing personal emotions is particularly salient when working with children who might have been maltreated. Personal experience of abuse can affect the perceptions professionals have and the conclusions they reach when evaluating what children say. Goodman *et al* (2002) found that professionals with personal experience of childhood abuse were more likely to rate children's statements as being suggestive of abuse, when in fact the children had not been abused, than colleagues who had not suffered abuse during their childhood.

The literature on interviewing children, for example in child and adolescent mental health, has emphasised the importance of the professionals' own behaviour and how these adults manage their own thoughts, emotions and biases (e.g. Angold, 1994). Studies that have looked at style and approach have found that interviews that were 'driven' by the professional, and those in which the pace and agenda were the practitioner's rather than the child's and which were accompanied by a hectoring tone, resulted in much greater error.

Ceci & Bruck's (1995) critique of overtly poor interviewing of younger children in the USA emphasised the central importance of interviewer behaviour, preconception and expressed emotion. They analysed the effect of overtly leading questions, repeated questioning and lack of appropriate recording of interviews in the genesis of misinformation. These authors present a compelling analysis to support the primary role of interviewer bias in the production of confusing or false accounts of maltreatment (Ceci & Bruck, 1995, pp. 79–105).

Issues such as the ones briefly referred to above are relatively neglected in the guidelines that are available to assist practitioners working with children in these situations. Active work on interviewer bias appears rarely in training programmes, either at an introductory or at an advanced stage (Davies *et al*, 1998). This may be because such matters are seen to be self-evident. However, it is very clear from examination of high-profile cases (Butler-Sloss, 1988; Clyde, 1992; Ceci & Bruck, 1995), as well as from the evaluation of routine interview practice with allegedly sexually abused children in the field (Lamb *et al*, 1999), that practitioners ignore or at least do not always apply these lessons. Hence they are stressed here and it is suggested that they be accorded at least equal weight to the verbal content of assessments.

## Bias among practitioners

There are two principal types of bias that are of importance to this field. The first is expectancy, and the second is typecasting (the former has been termed 'confirmatory bias' and the latter 'the representativeness heuristic').

*Expectancy* involves the practitioner placing greater weight and importance on things that the child communicates that fit in with the practitioner's expectations For example, a practitioner, hearing from a child that she does not like having a shower at daddy's house, forms a premature conclusion that this implies sexual abuse. Another example might be a practitioner assuming that inter-parental violence has occurred when a child relays an account in school of daddy hitting mummy. In both examples violence may have occurred, but there could be several other explanations for the child's utterances.

*Typecasting* refers to the professional prematurely or mistakenly placing the child within a certain category of children, and this leads the practitioner to presuppose that this particular child shares characteristics with the group in question. For example, a practitioner concluded, when faced with a child who appeared reluctant and embarrassed to communicate, that there was a sexual abuse ring in existence. This was in the context of another child having shown severe anxiety symptoms within the same class, who had talked about his teacher in very negative and sexualised terms. Another example involved a child with an unexplained bruise who expressed positive allegiance to his mother and new cohabitee. The practitioner jumped to the conclusion that this was an example of a physically abused child demonstrating an abnormal degree of loyalty to his abusive parents. As in the first example, the practitioner's assumptions were feasible, but other possibilities existed and there was danger in coming to premature conclusions.

Jones, D. P. H. (2003) *Communicating with Vulnerable Children*. London: Gaskell.

Ceci & Bruck (1995) point out that in situations where the practitioner's bias turns out in fact to be correct, bias proves to be a characteristic that results in a greater amount of information being revealed by the child. On the other hand, if the professional is incorrect in an assumption, the child makes errors of commission (in experimental studies). This is an extremely important observation because biased practitioners therefore obtain positive reinforcement and personal reward from their biased views and practices when they meet children who have been abused and where their assumptions are correct. They are therefore able to demonstrate great skill to their colleagues and bask in the false conclusion that their approaches and techniques are highly developed, and moreover effective in obtaining 'disclosures'. However, it is the very same interviewers who are the ones most prone to produce erroneous accounts from children who have *not* been abused (i.e. who do not fit the professional's stereotype or bias). These errors are, of course, filtered out and even unknown to practitioners who maintain these kinds of bias.

Bias may be conveyed to the child either verbally or non-verbally. Practitioners may directly express their views, attitudes and presumptions. Bias may be conveyed indirectly by practitioners through things said, or omitted, by their expression of emotion, or through their level of interest in selected parts of the child's account. It is important to remember that children who have been abused are more likely to be sensitised to the expressed emotions of adults who surround them. Thus, interviewer distress can often lead to children deciding not to reveal information (Wade & Westcott, 1997). In contrast, a child who has been subject to neglect may well be persuaded by the practitioner's interest and warm concern to go along with a particular line of questioning, in order to retain the professional's interest for longer.

# Technique

Technique involves the use of techniques that are more likely to lead to accurate and complete accounts, while avoiding those that are more prone to errors of omission or commission. Thus methods of communication that encourage free recall from the child and those associated with the highest levels of accuracy are preferred. Some techniques are known to be potentially inaccurate and in general should be avoided. These include the use of leading or suggestive comments to the child, the making of evaluative comments, and calls upon the child to imagine or pretend in order to clarify facts (whereas asking a child to imagine or pretend is appropriate if the practitioner is seeking to elicit feelings or emotions). The use of specific techniques such as anatomically detailed dolls is much more controversial.

The advantages and disadvantages of their use are discussed in Chapter 12.

It is clearly not appropriate to employ undue pressure and coercion when communicating with children. This can range from overt harassment and persistent questioning with an obvious intention to extract disclosure of abuse from a child, through to subtler means of pressurising a child, either verbally or through expressed emotion, to guide the child in a predetermined direction. It is important to recognise that interviewers may be wholly unaware that they are doing this, and indeed be both resistant and horrified when their own practices are subjected to scrutiny. It has long been known that the mere selective attentiveness or change in interest level of the interviewer, in response to different parts of the child's account, are detected and understood by the child, and this, in turn, can affect the accuracy of an account. Thus compliant children, and younger children as well as those with learning disabilities, may be especially prone progressively to adapt their account in response to the interviewer's subtle cues of encouragement. These may be non-verbal cues, or consist of simple verbal encouragement in response to items that the interviewer expects or wishes to hear, contrasted with silence or relative disinterest for those items regarded as unimportant. For example, the author has seen interviews in which a succession of subtle verbal and non-verbal signs of encouragement followed any small sexual disclosure that the child made, while the child's descriptions of physically abusive acts perpetrated upon him, as well as incidents of inter-parental violence, were met with distinct indifference. The result was that the child offered no further information about the acts of physical violence, while at the same time appearing to elaborate on sexual matters. If this were to be repeated several times in the interview, or over repeated interview sessions, it is easy to see how false or at least confusing accounts might emerge.

Overtly coercive interviewing is associated with police interviewing of crime suspects, in the days before codes of good practice as to the appropriate way of obtaining information (Mortimer & Shepherd, 1999). While such techniques may be disappearing fast, it can be salutary for the interviewer to consider why and in what way such techniques lead to error. The criticisms levelled at children's interviewing in high-profile child abuse cases have involved social workers and mental health professionals as well as police officers undertaking what would be considered coercive practices.

For these reasons consensus groups discourage selective reinforcement, for example rewarding the child with verbal compliments, such as 'well done', 'that's good' or 'good boy'. The more overt practice of promising rewards in the future in return for a 'disclosure' now – for example 'When you've told me about what daddy did to you then we can have a break and a drink' – should not be used.

# Implications for the practitioner

The core skills and qualities set out in this chapter are required by all those who communicate with children, whatever the primary purpose of the interaction. However, the importance of having these skills and qualities is brought into sharp relief by the demands of communicating with children who have experienced adverse events. The sensitivities of this group of children to the communications of adult professionals are likely to be greater than those of other children. At the same time, good communication skills on the part of the professional are desperately needed by children who have been victimised, in order to allow them to impart any information or express their concerns. Equally, the potential consequences of poorly developed professional skills are serious for such children, as they can lead to erroneous accounts and distortions of children's memories (Oates *et al*, 2000). Inadequate skill levels are liable to produce not only errors of commission (false positive accounts of abuse or maltreatment from children) but also errors of omission (in which a compromised child may be left unheard and unprotected). The consequences can be serious, psychosocially, emotionally and legally (see Chapter 4).

# Summary

The professional approach necessary for communicating with children can be summarised in terms of those qualities more likely to lead to positive outcomes, on the one hand, and those to avoid, on the other. They are as follows:

## *Positive professional qualities*

- Listen to and understand the child.
- Convey genuine empathic concern, to a degree that is congruent with the child or young person's situation.
- Adopt the perspective that it is the child or young person who is the expert, not the adult.
- Allow children to freely recall their experiences.
- Maintain neutrality and self-management.
- Operate within a context of continuing professional development and critical review of practice. When undertaking *initial assessments* (Department of Health *et al*, 2000), the following should be added:
  - Identify the aims of the work, including who has asked for the assessment and what plans have been decided upon, and why.
  - Record the exchange, including both its content and duration.
  - Clarify any ambiguous communication arising from the child or adult.

- Report the content of communications afterwards, as appropriate, to any other agency or group of professionals, having obtained the necessary consent to do so.

## Qualities to avoid or discourage

- Maintaining assumptions or biased views that may influence the interchange between the child and adult.
- Employing leading questions or other techniques that are prone to error.
- Using coercion and pressurising methods of enquiry.

# CHAPTER 7

# How concerns come to professional attention: the context for practice

How and to whom do children who have been victimised or exposed to negative life events communicate their experiences? Understanding these issues is an essential basis for professional practice.

Children and young people experience a wide variety of negative events and situations that may lead to their being harmed physically or psychologically. Not all of these are readily appreciated by the child as harmful; and even if they are experienced negatively, not all children wish to speak about them, or know who to tell about them. Children and young people choose whether to communicate. However, younger children cannot choose so readily, because either their understanding or their language is more limited, or because of absence of opportunity, personal confidence or sufficient trust to tell another what is on their mind. Some children are fearful of communicating their experiences, while others may have been actively inhibited from doing so. Equally, the other side of the equation is the recipient's response or lack of it. Not all the children or adults to whom the child first communicates will respond in such a way as to lead to relief or protection.

## Use and misuse of the term 'disclosure'

Critics have argued that the term 'disclosure' should be jettisoned because it is imprecise and is associated with stereotypical views about children's gradual unfolding of concerns over time. The various meanings and ideas associated with the term 'disclosure' are described here.

One use is to describe the process that occurs between experiencing a traumatic event and communicating that experience to another person. Sometimes the term is restricted to communication of such events to a professional person, but more frequently abuse is revealed to a friend or family member, rather than a professional. The communication may not be direct, or indeed intended. For example, some children display unusually sexualised behaviour and, because of this, others become suspicious about the possibility of sexual abuse having occurred. In other cases sexual abuse of the child is witnessed, and so not

Jones, D. P. H. (2003) *Communicating with Vulnerable Children*. London: Gaskell.

**73**

deliberately disclosed. Use of the term 'disclosure' is usually, therefore, restricted to those children who talk about abuse that has occurred to them or, in the case of children with specific impairments of communication or language, otherwise specifically communicate their experience. There has been considerable debate as to whether this process of disclosure is typically an extended one or not (Bradley & Wood, 1996; Jones, 1996) and we return to this issue below.

Disclosure has also been used to describe the proportion of investigative interviews with children suspected of having been abused that result in clear accounts emerging from the children. This is a very specific use of the term, which focuses on a narrower time band in the child's life than the overall process of revelation from occurrence to communicating that fact to others.

Disclosure has also been used to describe interviewing practice that is specifically designed to overcome the presumed obstacles that a child has to communicating abusive experiences. In this sense, the term 'disclosure interview' has been used. This is clearly presumptive and associated with interview practice that sets out to confirm an existing idea that the child has been abused (Ceci & Bruck, 1995; Jones, 1996; Poole & Lamb, 1998).

Disclosure will not be used in that sense in this text, but where it is used it will refer to the process, from the child's perspective, of communication of events that have been experienced. It will be restricted to direct communications (either verbal or in another form if that is the child's principal way of communicating).

So what factors are relevant to the presentation of concerns by children? What are the processes involved and which factors facilitate or impede presentation to professionals? The areas listed below inform our understanding of whether, and if so how, a particular child will be likely to communicate experience of negative life events.

- Developmental considerations.
- Social and emotional factors.
- Children at different stages in the child protection system.
- Children's presentations of sexual abuse allegations.
- Children's accounts subsequent to discovery of physical harm.
- Qualitative studies of children's experiences of telling others.
- Adult recollections of childhood abuse.
- Delay in disclosing adverse experiences.
- Have sexual assault prevention programmes affected presentation of concerns?

The factors that may affect a child's ability or willingness to communicate experiences to others are then summarised.

It should be noted that most of the information in this area relates to child sexual abuse – there is much less work in the field of physical abuse, or issues such as children's observation of domestic violence and other adversities (Kolko *et al*, 1996).

## Developmental considerations

Age and development will affect children's capacity to describe their experiences (Davies & Westcott, 1998). Several aspects and combinations of developmental maturation are likely to be relevant in this respect:

- Children's capacity to understand their world and their role within it.
- Their capacity to understand the nature and meaning of the complexity of adult behaviours, such as sexual abuse or inter-parental violence.
- Their ability to realise that they are being subjected to acts that the majority of people would consider wrong, or that they are being exploited or abused by an adult.
- Their degree of maturity in terms of language and communication.
- Their memory abilities.

Young children, for example below the age of four years, may have insufficient knowledge of the world to understand that they are being subjected to harm. This could affect children in two different ways. It may lead some children to be unaffected by embarrassment or concern that they have been subjected to wrong or immoral activities, which could render them less inhibited about describing their experiences. On the other hand, because of a lack of understanding, they may not appreciate that there are being subjected to harm or exploitation, which would render them less likely to disclose that experience to anyone else.

Retrospective accounts by older children and adults suggests that at least some children are reluctant to describe their experiences because they do not fully understand or are perplexed about the normality or otherwise of personal experiences and harm in childhood. Children under the age of seven years have difficulty understanding their own role in and responsibility for what happens to them. This sometimes leads to what has been described as 'egocentricity' on the part of younger children, which may in turn lead them to feeling responsible for things that have been done to them (Cicchetti, 1989). Furthermore, young children's underdeveloped ability to communicate in words and concepts that can be understood by adults may further hamper their capacity to tell others about their experiences.

This problem is compounded if the boundaries of intimate care have been gradually breached over time. For example, it is known that some sexual abuse begins with activities that are barely distinguishable from general expressions of affection or bathing, toileting or intimate care. Over time, the actions become more overtly sexual in nature, but for younger children this gradual process can be difficult to appreciate and thereby problematic to communicate. This process is thought to be particularly difficult for children with learning disabilities or communication impairments (see Chapter 5, and Westcott & Jones, 1999).

Some children and adults, looking back on when they were younger, describe complex interactions between their relative developmental immaturity, sense of right and wrong, peer relationships and their willingness to describe unpleasant experiences. However, we do not know for how many children these issues pose difficulties. Some children, at any rate, describe negative experiences without such difficulties (Bradley & Wood, 1996). We do not know what distinguishes those children who can describe unpleasant experiences from those who appear to have more difficulty. Are they, for example, of a different temperament or more securely attached to their parents? There is some suggestion, at least within the field of child sexual abuse, that the closer the relationship between the child and the abuser, the less likely the child is freely to describe the abusive experiences (see below).

Children under the age of five years have more immature memory systems than older children (see Chapter 2). They register less, have more problems with retrieval and forget more quickly than older children. Their immature memories are also more susceptible to suggestive influences. These qualities render younger children at greater disadvantage subsequently, when describing their experiences to adults.

## Social and emotional factors

Social and emotional factors also affect children of different ages in different ways. The disclosing of noxious events may be inhibited by the child's sense of embarrassment, guilt and fear. These factors are heightened in the case of sexual adversity (see below). In experimental studies, embarrassment over genital touching had a greater inhibitory effect on children as they got older. In one study, children over the age of six years or so, perhaps because they were embarrassed about the social implications of genital touching, appeared to be inhibited from disclosing this information to an adult (Saywitz *et al*, 1991). In the same study, younger children, under the age of five, were much less inhibited, possibly because they did not have the same sense of personal embarrassment.

Not all sexual abuse is accompanied by the induction of guilt, or coercion or threats, but a substantial proportion is. What is not clear is how such coercion affects children's disclosure of information. In some studies offender threats did not substantially influence the likelihood of disclosure (Sauzier *et al*, 1989). However, in a study of children where sexual abuse had been alleged and they were witnesses in the criminal prosecution of their abuser, threats and the child's constant fear did have an influence on disclosure (Goodman *et al*, 1992; Goodman-Brown *et al*, 2003). Overall, it appears that embarrassment may affect some children's capacity to disclose sexual or other forms of intimate abuse. In addition, although there is conflicting evidence concerning the influence of offender threats, it does seem that these inhibit some children's disclosure of traumatic events.

The social support available to the child appears to influence disclosure. In both experimental studies (Moston & Egleberg, 1992) and studies of sexually abused children (Greenstock & Pipe, 1996), those who enjoyed greater social support from peers (Jones & Ramchandani, 1999) or parents appeared to find it easier to discuss intimate or traumatic events that they had experienced. It is likely that children who experience positive social support will have less fear about the negative consequences of disclosure, and also know that they will have a parent or friends' tolerance for such disclosure. This relationship was indeed found to be the case in one study that examined a range of factors that influenced how and why children told about their experiences of sexual abuse (Goodman-Brown *et al*, 2003).

## Children at different stages in the child protection system

We now consider the numbers of children who are within child welfare agency and police systems. We have some idea of the number of cases referred to public agencies because of suspected harm in Western countries. The annual incidence of sexual abuse based on Child Protection Agency reports in the USA is approximately 2 per 1000 children. However, this figure differs from the community-based figures by a factor of three. That is, only about a third of sexual abuse cases come to the attention of public agencies (Finkelhor, 1994). Those that do are more likely to include penetrative or orogenital contact.

Approximately half of the cases referred to social services departments because of suspected sexual abuse in the USA and the UK are considered by that department to be confirmed cases of sexual abuse (see Chapter 3). In the other half there is a varied mixture of cases, ranging from malicious false allegations through to erroneous concerns made good faith, and another group where suspicion remains but conclusions cannot be reached in either direction (Jones & McGraw, 1987; Oates *et al*, 2000).

Not all the substantiated cases reach the family justice system, for a variety of reasons: some because the abuse is considered extra-familial; others because family court proceedings to ensure the welfare of the child are not considered either necessary or feasible to pursue. Hence only some of the cases referred to social services departments filter through to the family justice system. The number finding their way to the criminal justice system is smaller still and represent only a tiny proportion of the total number of cases of child abuse.

## Children's presentations of sexual abuse allegations

Some studies of children referred to public agencies because of suspected or actual abuse have described the way in which disclosure occurred. The majority of these show a wide variation in the timing of disclosure: some children tell about their abuse soon after the last time it occurred, whereas others take much longer. In addition, some disclosures are deliberate and others accidental. For example, in one study approximately three-quarters of pre-school children made accidental disclosures. In contrast, older children almost all made deliberate disclosures of abuse. That is, the older children talked about sexual abuse to an adult, whereas the younger children quite commonly displayed unusual behaviour or provided other indirect indications that led to adults' suspicion of abuse (Campis et al, 1993). In other studies, however, far greater proportions of pre-school children made verbal disclosures as opposed to indirect, or so-called accidental, ones (e.g., Mian et al, 1986).

Returning to the issue of timing, in one study, 42% of sexually abused children involved in the legal system had told someone about their abuse within 48 hours of the last occurrence (Goodman et al, 1992). A further 19% disclosed within the first month following the last assault, 14% delayed their disclosures for between one and six months, and 15% waited for more than six months (no information on remainder). Further analysis of the study data (Goodman-Brown et al, 2003) indicated that children feared negative consequences or harm to others or to themselves and that this inhibited their disclosure, and that young children were quicker to disclose abuse than were teenagers. Moreover, children abused within the family were less likely to tell than those abused extra-familially. In this study, gender did not influence whether the child told, but race did: Caucasian children took longer to disclose than did Hispanic children, who in turn took longer than Afro-American children (independent of socio-economic status). Interestingly, maternal support and parental emotional health did not significantly relate to children's disclosures. However, children who felt responsible for the abuse took far longer to disclose (Goodman-Brown et al, 2003). These results have been described in some detail here in order to illustrate the influence of a wide range of different factors on the process of disclosure.

# Children's accounts subsequent to discovery of physical harm

A significant proportion of children do not disclose the abuse that medical evidence strongly suggests has taken place, for example where there is medical evidence of venereal disease, or where physically abused children have been asked how their injuries occurred (Lawson & Chaffin, 1992; Kolko, 2002).

# Qualitative studies of children's experiences of telling others

There have been few studies of children's own experiences of trying to bring their plight to the attention of others. What does emerge from the findings, nonetheless, is that many children felt under intense pressure before having first spoken out about abuse. Sometimes this pressure came from within, due to feelings of embarrassment, guilt or shame, while for others it was an external pressure from the abuser, indirectly or directly. Often both these sets of pressures combined to prevent the child telling anyone until the child finally 'cracked'. Some describe telling a friend, others a parent and others a teacher, but usually without any clear objective in mind other than simply talking about something that had become intolerable or that was distressing (Prior *et al*, 1994; Berliner & Conte, 1995; Sharland *et al*, 1996; Wade & Westcott, 1997).

# Adult recollections of childhood abuse

A further source of information is studies of adults recalling their childhood experiences of abuse (e.g., Anderson *et al*, 1993; Fleming, 1997). These are usually sexual experiences and the definition of what constitutes abuse varies. Some studies include exposure and attempted touching, while others restrict the definition to touching genitalia or penetrative abuse. Combining the results of several large-scale studies, the prevalence of child sexual abuse is estimated at between 15% and 30% for females, and between 5% and 15% for males (Fergusson & Mullen, 1999; Jones, 2000b).

It has been estimated that less than 10% of sexual abuse revealed in these adult surveys was made known to official agencies at the time of abuse, during childhood (Fergusson & Mullen, 1999). Slightly more was reported to parents or other adults at the time but not made known to child welfare or law enforcement authorities (Fergusson & Mullen, 1999). In one study of adults recalling childhood experiences only 39%

had told anyone about their experience of sexual abuse within a year of its occurrence (Finkelhor, 1984). Once again, this suggests that reluctance to disclose is a significant feature of child sexual abuse.

There is considerably less evidence about physical abuse or other adversities, although under-reporting during childhood has emerged from the long-term studies of adults remembering childhood mal-treatment (Prescott *et al*, 2000), as well as from studies of children who have witnessed other forms of intra-familial violence (Kolko *et al*, 1996).

## Delay in disclosing adverse experiences

The studies described above suggest that, for most children at any rate, delay and reluctance to describe unpleasant events are to be expected, especially for sexual experiences in childhood. Summit (1983), in a highly influential article, described an accommodation syndrome, based on his clinical work with adults who had been sexually abused in childhood. In this syndrome, children who had been sexually abused adapted to their plight, gradually disclosing their situation, only for some to retract their accounts when met by subsequent disbelief among the adults they encountered. Several years later this was challenged by Bradley & Wood (1996), who reported that the majority of children in their study of children who were alleging sexual abuse described their experiences without such hesitation. They therefore challenged the prevailing view (Jones, 2000a). However, it should be noted that the children in Bradley & Wood's study had already disclosed to someone. The difference between these two viewpoints may underline the need to consider the entire time-line, from the child's initial experience of unpleasant events through to the child describing it to an adult who can intervene. Between these two poles many things can happen, and it seems likely that the course or trajectory is different for different children.

Smith *et al* (2000) reported the results from the National Women's Study in the USA, which has shed light on this important area. The advantage of their study is that it was based on a non-clinical, population sample, rather than on a selected sample of students or clinically referred people. They found that 28% of the 288 women who had retrospectively reported sexual abuse experienced before their eighteenth birthday had never told anyone about that experience until the research interview. Overall, a quarter of their sample had told someone within a month of the event occurring, with the remainder delaying disclosure over a varying period of time. They found that abuse by a stranger, or single events, were more likely to be reported rapidly. However, those with a family relationship with the perpetrator, or who were younger when abused, were much more likely to delay disclosure

Jones, D. P. H. (2003) *Communicating with Vulnerable Children*. London: Gaskell.

past one month, or to not tell anyone until the research interviews. Interestingly, threats, force, injury to the victim, use of a weapon and the severity of the abuse itself were unrelated to whether the disclosure was delayed or rapid.

## Have sexual assault prevention programmes affected the presentation of concerns?

Smith *et al*'s (2000) study involved adults who, as children, had not generally been influenced by the sort of education programmes that became common in the USA during the 1980s. The authors did find, however, that the younger women in their sample appeared to be more likely to report childhood experiences of sexual abuse than older women. Nevertheless, the overall rate of disclosure was still low and disclosure was delayed for many of the victims. Thus, it may be that we can understand more about the process of presentation from studies that have examined the impact of prevention programmes.

MacIntyre & Carr (1999) explored the impact of the 'Stay Safe' programme in Ireland. They compared the rate of referral for suspected sexual abuse before and after the introduction of that prevention programme, in one of the few studies of its kind. They found that there was a higher rate of initial disclosure in those children who had participated in the programme, and that these disclosures were more likely to be made to the children's teachers than they were before the programme's introduction. Furthermore, the rate of confirmed abuse was greater among the participants than in the comparison group. The children were also more likely to communicate their concerns deliberately than they were previously. It will, of course, be many years before we know for certain what impact prevention programmes have on disclosure rates. It is quite possible that the combination of prevention programmes and a greater willingness among the general population to acknowledge the existence of family violence and child maltreatment will lead to reduced secrecy. However, it seems unlikely that these influences alone will be powerful enough to counter those forces that conspire to delay disclosure of unpleasant events for many children.

## Summary

There is no typical pattern that describes how children communicate unpleasant or harmful events to adults. What is clear from the studies reviewed above is that there is wide variation. While some children delay their communications, others rapidly disclose their concerns. Broadly there are four groups of children who have experienced harm: those who do not communicate their experiences; those who make partial communications; those who clearly communicate to a parent or a professional other than a social worker or police officer; and those who make direct and clear communication about their concerns to a professional from an official agency such as the police, a social work department or the National Society for the Prevention of Cruelty to Children (NSPCC).

Not all clear communications find their way to official child welfare or law enforcement systems, even when a child describes abuse or other serious harm. We know this from studies of adults recalling their childhood experiences. It may be thought that studies of adults will relate only to a time when there was less general awareness of the problems of child abuse and neglect and when systems and procedures of child protection had not yet developed fully. However, studies of the reporting system within the USA (where reporting of child abuse and neglect concerns is required by law) reveal that a substantial proportion of known abuse is still not referred to the welfare or law enforcement systems.

Thus, only a proportion of children's concerns find their way through to official child welfare or law enforcement systems. Some parents, for example, take immediate steps to protect their child, and ensure that there will never be any further contact with the abuser, yet do not report the situation to professionals. We do not know all the reasons for this, but from what little information is available, fear of the consequences of disclosure to public agencies and the family disruption that would follow appear to be the most common reasons. However, adults recalling childhood experiences have not always been able to discover why their parents, or other adults, decided not to relay their experiences to official agencies.

So, what is known about children who, for one reason or another, do not communicate serious concerns to others? This is clearly a difficult area to study contemporaneously. Potential sources of information are clinical studies of children in compromised situations through child abuse and neglect, or of those observing or knowing about their parents' violent behaviour towards one another, or of those living with a parent who poses a threat to the child's welfare through substance misuse. Another source of information is adults recalling their childhood and trying to remember why they delayed telling anyone about their plight. From these studies the following groups of reasons for delay emerge:

- The child's lack of understanding.
- Fear or embarrassment.
- Adult influence and requirements for secrecy.
- Pressures related to relationships or attachments to significant others.

- Choice based on weighing the alternatives.
- Lack of sufficient trust or opportunity to communicate.
- Psychological condition of the child.

This summary of those factors that are pertinent to how concerns come to be presented can contribute to professional practice. It informs many of the practice suggestions that follow in the next chapters. Victimised children present their concerns to adults in various ways. It is probable that those who have not been so clearly victimised, but nonetheless were exposed to considerable adversity, have a similarly wide range of ways in which their concerns are presented. Equally clear is that the responses and receptiveness of the adults whom they 'tell' can vary from the sensitive and effective to minimisation and denial. It seems that a significant minority of victimised children do not communicate their experiences to anyone.

Subsequent chapters will now consider best practice with respect to children who do present to professionals, whether tentatively or more directly.

# Part II

# Practice issues

The chapters in Part II are concerned with practice. They contain summaries of policy considerations, the available evidence and recommendations for practitioners. Part II starts with an orientation to the different settings and types of professional to whom a child may turn. Chapters 9–11 describe the different contexts for communication with children. Non-verbal and indirect communication is reviewed in Chapter 12, and advice for parents in Chapter 13. Part II ends with a chapter that presents a framework with which to analyse information, and reviews training implications and future directions for research.

Jones, D. P. H. (2003) *Communicating with Vulnerable Children*. London: Gaskell.

**85**

# CHAPTER 8

# Practice issues: introduction

Communication with children extends beyond talking alone. The government's assessment framework (Department of Health *et al*, 2000) emphasises this in its paragraphs entitled 'Communicating with Children' (3.41–3.45). The following five critical components are described: seeing, observing, engaging, talking, and doing activities with children. All those who work with children are in a position to do any one of these, or combinations thereof. Hence, although in this book we will refer primarily to talking to children, components of the other four elements described in the assessment framework will be part of the practitioner's work.

Children communicate adverse experiences in various ways and at different points during their childhood (see Chapter 7). Some children's concerns are presented unambiguously and lead to their assessment by a relevant professional. Others are less well defined. In general, children who have experienced specific traumatic events or losses in their life are more likely to show non-specific emotional and behavioural difficulties than discrete indicators of a particular trauma. Hence the search for explicit 'indicators' of particular experiences is likely to be fruitless. Furthermore, when children start to talk about their experiences, or indirectly raise concerns, it may be to a variety of adults: parents, carers or professionals.

Anyone working with children and adolescents can therefore be faced with a child who wants to communicate distress. This applies to the busy teacher, health visitor, general practitioner, youth worker, parent or other carers and voluntary workers. For some professionals it is a relatively frequent event, for example teachers (MacIntyre & Carr, 1999). Children spend a great deal of their time in school and develop trust in their teachers. Teachers are often the first adults outside the home with whom a child forms a relationship.

Sometimes it is already known that a child is in difficult circumstances. Children in such circumstances may include those not living in their own homes, those being looked after by local authority social services departments, those coming from homes where there is significant disruption or even violence, and children of divorcing or separating parents. For other children traumatic events are more obvious, such as children who have witnessed a house fire, an assault or even murder.

Often, however, no such prior knowledge exists and it is the child's manner that changes inexplicably or communicates something unusual, indicative or concerning to the professional. Chapter 9 is directed at these kinds of situations. Its aim is to provide guidance on those first responses to children's concerns, for any practitioner who is presented with a child who wants to talk about adverse experiences.

Chapter 10 is concerned with meetings and communications with children as part of an established assessment process. One such example is the meeting with the child that forms part of an initial assessment led by a social services department when it has been referred a potential child in need. This includes children who are referred because their health or development may be impaired without the provision of support or services, because they are disabled or because they may be suffering or at risk of suffering significant harm (collectively known as 'children in need') (Department of Health *et al*, 1999, paras 5.5, 5.6, 5.13; Department of Health *et al*, 2000, chapter 3).

Professionals other than social workers undertake assessments. Examples include those working in child and adolescent mental health services, those working in services for children with learning disabilities and children's guardians. Here, too, seeing, observing, engaging, talking and undertaking activities with children form an established part of the assessment processes. These meetings with children are not confined to enquiries about possible adverse events, but have the broader purpose of understanding, from the child's perspective, what is the nature of the presenting problem, and what factors may be helpful in understanding and responding to it, by the particular service. Enquiry about possible adverse experiences may therefore form part of the initial assessment processes of a range of professionals.

In-depth interviews are covered in Chapter 11. They are interviews with children where there are particular concerns about their welfare, sufficient to have led to a referral to social services, and where a core assessment is being undertaken. These children are principally those suspected of suffering or likely to be suffering significant harm (Section 47 enquiries – see Department of Health *et al*, 1999, sections 5.33—5.38; Department of Health *et al*, 2000, paras 3.15–3.19). In some instances, there will be clear evidence that a crime has taken place; this will require an investigative interview in order to gather evidence for possible criminal proceedings. *Achieving Best Evidence* (Home Office *et al*, 2002) should be followed as the appropriate guide for such interviews (Department of Health *et al*, 1999, paras 5.39–5.41).

However, many situations are not so clear-cut. After initial intake and assessment there may be no evidence that would result in a decision to undertake an investigative interview, or it may be decided that an investigative interview is not indicated for the present. The primary focus then becomes an assessment of the child's needs. A

Jones, D. P. H. (2003) *Communicating with Vulnerable Children*. London: Gaskell.

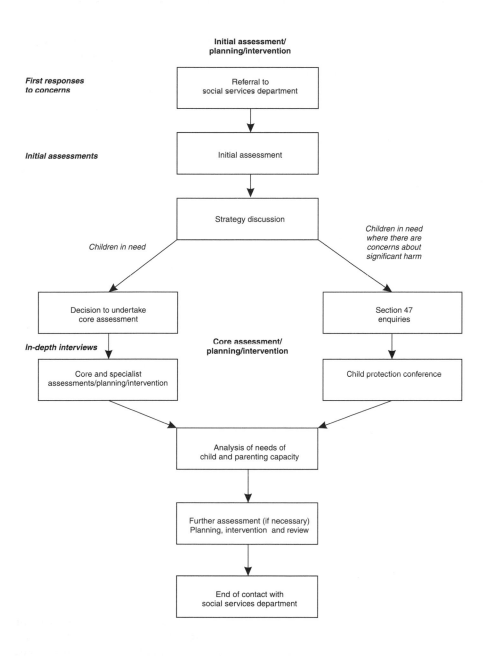

**Initial assessment/
planning/intervention**

*First responses
to concerns*

Referral to
social services department

*Initial assessments*

Initial assessment

Strategy discussion

*Children in need*

*Children in need
where there are
concerns about
significant harm*

Decision to undertake
core assessment

Section 47
enquiries

*In-depth interviews*

**Core assessment/
planning/intervention**

Core and specialist
assessments/planning/intervention

Child protection conference

Analysis of needs of
child and parenting capacity

Further assessment (if necessary)
Planning, intervention and review

End of contact with
social services department

**Figure 8.1** The assessment process and different kinds of communication with children.
(Adapted with permission from Department of Health *et al*, 2000, p. 33.)

component, but not the entirety, of that assessment of need will focus on whether the child has experienced adversity. Chapter 11 focuses on the assessment of this possibility.

Thus Chapters 9–11 deal respectively with talking to the child, initial assessment and in-depth interviews. The place of these three types of communication in relation to the process of assessment recommended by the government is represented in Figure 8.1. The three types of communication described in Chapters 9–11 have been superimposed upon the flowchart of the assessment process, in order to orientate the practitioner to the suggested use of these chapters.

Chapter 12, Indirect and non-verbal approaches, considers the major contribution that observation of children can make, as well as a discussion on the use of toys and drawing materials when communicating with children. Lastly, Chapter 13 gives guidance on advice for parents. In the past, parents have reported that they do not know how to respond to their child's concerns or how they should react to any subsequent concerns emerging after there has been an initial meeting or assessment of the child. Chapter 13 gives practitioners access to advice for parents who seek or require it.

Inevitably, there is some overlap between the chapters in Part II of the book, while at the same time not every eventuality can be covered. Nonetheless, the discussion and suggestions that follow convey the principles of accepted good practice, and these can be applied to the vast majority of situations encountered. The material is presented in terms of the principles and choices for interviewers rather than a schema of interviewing to be rigidly applied. This is partly because the approaches set out in Chapters 9 and 10 fall short of what might be termed an 'interview', but are briefer aspects of a broader enquiry. Chapter 11 deals with assessments that are more recognisable as an interview format, but even here the assessment may form part of a wider enquiry, rather than an interview that is solely concerned with whether the child has experienced adversity. A related reason for not recommending a rigid protocol is that it is intended that the approaches that follow be incorporated within a practitioner's existing assessment schema rather than be stand-alone.

Jones, D. P. H. (2003) *Communicating with Vulnerable Children*. London: Gaskell.

# CHAPTER 9

# Talking with the child: first responses to children's concerns

Any professional working with children can be faced with the situation where either a child wants to communicate or the professional needs to respond to a concern. Many of these situations are initiated by the child and emerge during the context of providing everyday services for children. A few examples illustrate the situations affecting different professionals:

A six-year-old girl tells her teacher that she does not want to go home with her mother's boyfriend (who has recently begun collecting her after school).

An eight-year-old boy is brought to his general practitioner complaining that his anal area is sore and has on one occasion bled after defecation.

A seven-year-old girl tells her friend that she does not like the baby-sitter (a boy of 16 who regularly sits for the child and her sister).

A seven-year-old girl complains to her social worker that she does not like it when her cousin comes to stay.

An 11-year-old girl says that she is worried about her mum having to go to the doctors because she has fallen downstairs again.

A six-year-old girl asks her teacher very anxiously who is collecting her from school today.

A four-year-old child is found on a routine examination by her health visitor to have unexplained bruises on the back of her legs.

An 11-year-old child becomes suddenly upset during school lessons, tearful and easily distressed, in marked change from her previous demeanour.

A 12-year-old girl shows a sudden deterioration in her schoolwork combined with reduced concentration and a tendency towards frequent daydreaming.

A 14-year-old boy tells his teacher that he is very worried about his parents' divorce and the fact that his father drinks to excess and sometimes pushes his mother around.

A 16-year-old girl tells her classmate that her boyfriend is regularly assaulting her. The friend tells her mother.

A 14-year-old runs away from home and finds sanctuary with another family, whose daughter is the same age. While there she talks to her friend about conflict within her family. The friend tells her mother, who contacts social services.

A 13-year-old girl is admitted to the accident and emergency department of the local hospital because of alcohol intoxication and says that she does not wish to return home because she fears that her stepfather will be angry with her.

The professional who is in immediate contact with the child in situations such as those above would normally talk a little more with the child first to see what response, if any, is necessary. The four-year-old with bruising could be an exception, but even in these circumstances the practitioner would probably want to talk to the parents first. These types of situation face a wide range of front-line professionals working with children. Policy issues are considered first in this chapter, then the research evidence, before turning to the implications of these for the practitioner.

## Policy and procedural issues

Guidance is available for professionals who become aware of indications of harm, or where physical signs of assault are evident. The professional is usually required to pass on the observation to a specified agency to make sure that a child's needs are responded to appropriately. For instance, once a professional such as a teacher, health visitor, doctor or youth worker becomes aware that a child may be in need of protection, or may have been subject to a criminal act, then the responsibility becomes clear to refer the child to the appropriate agency, namely the local social services department or the police (Department of Health *et al*, 1999). However, in the type of situation illustrated in the cameos above, the situation is much less clear. A response from the professional is necessary first, in order to see whether the case should be referred on or should remain within the professional's own agency, or whether no further action is required for the present. These first responses to the type of concerns illustrated above generally lie outside the remit of locally or nationally agreed procedures. Procedural guidance begins once professionals' first responses have already established the likelihood of abuse and generally advise the professional what to do next. So, what is known about these first responses?

It is clear that some professionals are reluctant to become involved with children's experiences. Some state their determination to focus on their perceptions of the limits and boundaries of their particular job, for example teachers who state that their job involves education only and that it is for others to deal with the child's welfare. Such reluctance can be understandable, because involvement in the child's welfare may demand time-consuming and potentially stressful communications with other agencies, parents and others. There has been little research on these issues, so their resolution must be sought from local policy combined with national law and guidance. Nonetheless, some relevant research evidence is available.

Research and audit on the use by various professionals of local child protection procedures has sometimes revealed surprisingly poor knowledge among professionals, with the exception of social workers. They are often poorly informed about: indicators of maltreatment or other traumas among children, local arrangements for referring concerns to other agencies, national guidance, and the roles of other professionals dealing with children in their geographical area. Hopefully the situation is improving, as multi-agency training initiatives have become more widespread. However, discussions involving multi-disciplinary groups during training have emphasised lack of mutual trust among professionals dealing with children, in addition to deficits in knowledge.

For some professionals (e.g. general practitioners, teachers), a perceived conflict of interest between their relationship and commitment to children and to their parents creates particular difficulties. Other professionals report dissatisfaction with the outcome of previous enquiries in relation to children considered to be at risk of harm. This has affected their willingness to refer their concerns in subsequent cases (Department of Health, 1995; Department of Health *et al*, 1999, para. 2.25). The evidence from enquiry reports consistently emphasises a lack of effective collaboration as a central issue when the reasons for the failure of professional systems to protect a child from serious abuse are explored retrospectively (Department of Health, 1991; Department of Health *et al*, 1999, paras 1.13, 2.25, 2.26.). Multi-disciplinary working involves human relationships between professionals, however, and not mere knowledge or familiarity with procedures or policies (Hudson, 2000).

In the USA, where reporting is a legal requirement, studies examining referrals made to designated professionals have consistently demonstrated that local professionals vary in their application of the law and some flout the rules, the potential consequences of non-reporting notwithstanding (Warner & Hansen, 1997).

It seems likely that the answer to these issues will rest with education and training initiatives, especially those that bring together diverse professionals into locally based discussion groups. Awareness-raising initiatives would seem sensible, too. Such approaches encourage debate, reflection and an appreciation of the perspective of other professionals, and these may improve levels of trust between individuals and groups. Although we do not have research evidence for its efficacy, locally based systems that provide advice and support for professionals who are concerned about a child's welfare, or face difficult dilemmas, appear to be a useful way forward.

## Consent

It is generally important to obtain informed consent from children and their parents in relation to any procedures that affect them (Department of Health *et al*, 1999; Department of Health, 2001; Tan & Jones, 2001). Younger children should be involved as far as possible and their assent or agreement sought, even if they are incapable of providing consent to examination or treatment (Tan & Jones, 2001). The communications described in this chapter are not formal 'interviews' but brief, frequently impromptu conversations instigated by the child or arising through the professional's normal work with the child. The purpose of the conversations is to see whether the child's welfare is being compromised. The professional does not know the answer to this question.

If there were clear-cut concerns about the child's safety, then referral to the appropriate agency would be the way forward. However, even in these circumstances the practitioner should seek permission from an adult with parental responsibility for referral to social services or others, unless to do so would place the child at risk of significant harm (Department of Health *et al*, 1999).

Overall, then, formal consent is not feasible or relevant to the initial responses to uncertain situations where the purpose of the practitioner's communication is to see whether there is cause for concern. If situations become more clear-cut, however, and it becomes evident that there should be professional concern about the child's welfare, or even safety, then in these circumstances the consent of the child and the parents should be sought, except when harm might result from doing so. When obtaining consent from parents, while legally it is only necessary to obtain consent from one parent who holds parental responsibility, if there is another who does, it is good practice to obtain theirs too. Currently, the threshold for dispensing with parental consent in order to talk with a child is set at the point where to seek consent would place the child at risk of significant harm (Department of Health *et al*, 1999). However, recommendation 65 of the *Victoria Climbie Inquiry* (Laming, 2003) suggests that this threshold should be lowered (for doctors and possibly other health professionals). At the time of writing, it is yet to be seen whether or not this recommendation is taken forward.

## Confidentiality

Requests for confidentiality are more likely to come from older children. The dilemma for the professional is that if concerns about the child's safety emerge, there will be an obligation to override requests for confidentiality. Where there are no such concerns the professional has greater discretion. Even in those circumstances where safety is an issue, the professional may be able to work with the child, to discuss the merits of referral over a period of time, particularly if safety is not a pressing concern. However, if the child is suffering or is likely to suffer significant harm, referral will be necessary and the confidentiality duties of the professional will need to come second to requirements to make sure the child is safe (Department of Health *et al*, 1999, paras 5.3–5.6).

## Research findings concerning first responses

The nature of these meetings has been little studied, except where criticisms have been made at the final outcome of a case, following an analysis of the initial reactions and responses to the child (Jones & McGraw, 1987; Ceci & Bruck, 1995). Nonetheless, several areas which are well understood can inform the basis for good practice at this point. These include: knowledge of what constitutes good communication skills with children (Chapter 6), an understanding of the predicament that children who have been victimised might be facing (Chapter 4), and research evidence on the negative consequences of early bias on the subsequent reliability of children's accounts (especially younger children and those with disabilities) (Chapters 2, 3, 5 and 6).

Field studies are difficult to conduct on the everyday conversations and communications of professionals such as teachers and health visitors. To date, field-based research has focused on substantive interviews with children who are suspected of having been abused (e.g. Lamb *et al*, 1998). The sessions were normally video-taped, audio-taped or at least systematically noted, and were conducted in very different circumstances from the type of communications discussed here. That is, the studies have involved children where there has been a substantial indication that they might have been abused and have therefore been brought to a specific investigative interview with a designated professional (normally a social worker or a police officer, or, in Israel, a youth examiner). There have been no studies of experimental communications either, because naturally these have, similarly, focused on simulated substantive communications and interviews with children concerning specific events, rather than the kind of response to non-specific concerns in everyday settings with which this chapter is concerned.

Good professional skills can help children who have had adverse experiences to find the means to communicate. However, not all children with concerns to convey will be able to trust a professional sufficiently to do so. In particular, children required to maintain secrecy, or those who have been threatened with severe consequences if they reveal the nature of their experiences, are likely to face a major dilemma.

It has been clinically observed that some children are exquisitely sensitive to the reactions and responses of adults. Studies of children who have experienced maltreatment suggest they are more likely than comparison children to be sensitive to adult responses (Sharland *et al*,

1996). We know that a significant proportion of children who are almost certain, medically, to have been subject to abuse are not able to communicate their predicament when formally interviewed about it (Lawson & Chaffin, 1992). It is clear that a great deal of this non-communication results from children's fear, embarrassment or feeling they will be not believed (Sharland *et al*, 1996). It is likely that some reticence also derives from the responses of the practitioner, particularly those who are not used to hearing about children's adverse experiences. However, practitioners' contributions to non-communication have not been systematically studied. We know from qualitative studies with children, looking back on their experiences of disclosure (see Chapter 7), that the sensitive responses of the first adults with whom they try to communicate are all-important. These are the very adults who are normally providing everyday, routine services for children and are not specifically trained to respond to children's concerns. Indeed, they often have no warning that a child wishes to communicate concerns until that child starts to do so. These are the teachers, doctors, health visitors, youth workers and others who are in the 'front line'.

There are no direct studies on the relationship between professionals' capacity to modulate or contain their emotional responses, such as shock, disgust, anger, horror or disbelief, and children's ability or willingness to communicate. However, studies that have asked children themselves, after they have communicated adverse experiences, can be revealing here. Children who have been studied after the event, when looking back at earlier opportunities to communicate their distress, generally say they were not given the opportunity or 'no one asked me'. Disabled children complain that the professional 'went too fast'. Whether at that earlier time a timely question or enquiry would have assisted such children is not known. When children describe why they chose a particular individual, they highlight general qualities in the professionals, such as the fact that they appeared interested, had time or that they seemed concerned, rather than the fact that they asked specific questions.

There is no systematic, prospective research available from field-based studies on the impact of initial communications on the subsequent accuracy of a child's accounts, where cases develop into enquiries about possible maltreatment. Thus, we do not know whether a focused or even a leading question from a professional, as part of a brief communication with a child, affects the subsequent process. It has been established that poor questioning and bias in *substantive* interviews with children affect accuracy, at least for some of the children who are questioned in this way (Ceci & Bruck, 1995). Also, studies that have looked at false reports (Jones & McGraw, 1987; Oates *et al*, 2000), court cases and judicial enquiries (Clyde, 1992) have traced the origin of spurious or erroneous accounts to poor questioning methods. In these explorations it appears that interviewer bias begins early on, and this applies to those everyday professionals who ask the first questions as well as the designated professionals who conduct later enquiries. By contrast, studies have shown that more accurate and complete accounts can be obtained from children in formal interviews where interviewer bias is deliberately reduced and the child positively encouraged to resist any suggestion emanating from the adult (Orbach *et al*, 2000).

Thus, while it is good practice to minimise closed or leading questions, we cannot assert that one or two inappropriate questions from a teacher or doctor have an effect on the entire subsequent course of events. On the contrary, the research evidence suggests that a more persistently biased atmosphere is required in order to create an erroneous account of maltreatment.

We know very little about how frequently particular professionals talk with children about adverse experiences. It seems probable that many such discussions do not lead to concerns about the child's overall welfare or require referral on. There is an urgent need for a variety of studies specifically focused on these communications and talks with children. Both field-based studies and experimental designs are required that can then be fed back to front-line practitioners working with children.

## Implications for practitioners

The key message from the foregoing is the importance of professionals conveying that they will listen and respond to the child. This can involve attention to non-verbal communication, so that the child appreciates that the professional is available, while at the same time not overpowering the child or in other ways leading the child to feel pressurised. This establishes a good basis for any subsequent action that may be necessary when responding to the child's needs.

All practitioners working with children can make themselves available to respond to concerns. Such professionals are often in a position of trust vis-à-vis children and therefore the ones to whom children turn in their search for a listening ear or for help. In addition, adverse experiences are likely to have an influence on the child's health, development or education and thus it is not surprising that teachers, doctors, health visitors, youth workers and others may need to identify and respond to children's concerns. While doing so, however, they must remain the teacher or health visitor, for this position will be essential in the future, whatever the child's current experience may be.

Teachers spend long periods of time on their own with children, that is without parents being present. They are also important figures with whom the children communicate and become attached, outside their home. Nonetheless, if children wish to communicate, they may find the presence of other children inhibiting, or find settings such as the head teacher's office associated with discipline or to be in other ways stigmatising. So it may be important for teachers to find an opportunity to communicate with them away from the main class group, yet in a setting that is sensitive to the child's individual situation.

Paediatricians and general practitioners normally see children together with their parents. Sometimes raising the issue of the child's possible reluctance with a parent and child together can allow a parent to withdraw temporarily if the child appears to want to communicate without the parent present.

As well as conveying a willingness to listen, the professional will often be able either to invite the child to elaborate on the matter that has just created the concern, or to see whether they would like to talk to a colleague. The approach will be open-ended and consist of an invitation to talk if the child so wishes. For example, children can be asked to say why they are concerned about a particular place or person (if they have just told the teacher about such a concern). A doctor or health visitor might be able to ask how the child got a sore, or bruise or mark. Or the child might be asked to say a bit more about an expressed worry. In all these situations specific questions are avoided and the question is phrased in an open-ended way without conveying either verbal or non-verbal presupposition about the basis for any concerns.

This may be difficult for professionals unused to exploring children's adverse experiences, particularly in circumstances where a series of non-specific indications have raised a teacher's or doctor's concerns over a period of time. It can sometimes be helpful for professionals to practise in their mind, or with colleagues, how they would respond to such situations, in order to refine their verbal and non-verbal responses. The importance of seeking help, support and advice from other colleagues cannot be stressed enough. For teachers this would probably involve discussion with the designated teacher within the school who has responsibility for children's pastoral issues and child protection matters. Similarly, for doctors and nurses, advice should be sought from the named or designated professional.

Exploring behavioural change can be difficult without suggestion. Asking to know more about sadness or apparent anxiety is relatively non-contentious. However, enquiring around behaviour and conduct change can be more difficult.

A five-year-old began to be very aggressive, and to hurt and distress other children in the playground. His teacher took him to one side and talked about the behaviour: 'We don't pinch and hit other children because they might get upset or hurt and that's why no one does that to you'. To which he replied, 'They do', in a sad and distressed manner. The teacher asked, 'Who does?', and discovered that the child's stepmother was apparently pinching and hitting him when he was naughty (which was very frequent) when alone in the house.

Jones, D. P. H. (2003) *Communicating with Vulnerable Children*. London: Gaskell.

The teacher discussed her concerns with the designated teacher for child protection matters within the school and between them they were able to help the stepmother to get professional help and support with managing his challenging behaviour. If the child had not spontaneously answered 'They do', it might have been appropriate for the teacher to ask directly 'Has anyone pinched or hit you like that?', without making reference to home or any particular place or person.

Suggestive practice by professionals could jeopardise future attempts to help and respond to the child's predicament. Poor practice can affect both decision making concerning the child's welfare and any potential criminal prosecution. By contrast, good practice at this stage lays the foundation for future work and helps establish children's trust in professionals as people who may be able to help, notwithstanding any ambivalent feelings they may have. Surveys of children and their immediate carers in the aftermath of investigations into suspected child abuse strongly underline the importance of these first communications, when children are taking their first tentative steps towards revealing sensitive matters (Roberts & Taylor, 1993; Prior *et al*, 1994; Sharland *et al*, 1996; Wade & Westcott, 1997).

It is important to record any conversation that raises a suspicion of abuse having occurred and to describe the setting in which the conversation occurred. The full sequence, including the professional's words as well as the child's, and a note about the non-verbal elements of communication, will be vitally important when it comes to subsequent evaluation and case planning. This record would normally be a written one, made as soon as possible after the communication has occurred. If any rough jottings were made during or immediately after the conversation, these should be kept, even if a fuller record is made in due course. This becomes especially important in those situations that progress to formal assessment procedures.

The front-line practitioner's next steps will now depend upon what, if anything, the child has said or otherwise indicated. The outcome of the professional's first response may be to reveal a hitherto unrecognised concern about the child's safety or, at the other end of the spectrum, concerns about the child being allayed. For some children the situation will remain unclear. In these circumstances it is important to keep a line of communication open with the child, while perhaps also arranging for other services to help respond to any needs for extra help the child may have. Further options include discussing the situation with a colleague, or seeking advice through the channels set out in local child protection procedures. It is important to avoid preventing children communicating if they appear to want to. This applies especially if the child is obviously describing very serious adverse events. The professional's role is simply to listen, make a note of the conversation and respond appropriately to the concerns that have arisen. If professionals are concerned about the child's safety, they should not attempt to investigate the situation independently, but instead arrange a referral to a designated child protection service for further action. Local procedures set out the referral routes to the social services department, the police or, in some areas, the NSPCC.

The front-line professionals' role is therefore limited to the first response, listening, making the appropriate record and arranging for the next steps to occur. However, the overall impression is that many professional concerns are allayed through such first responses, or alternatively a much lower level of need is identified, which then guides the most appropriate way forward. Overt child protection concerns are probably less frequently revealed.

Box 9.1 summarises the suggestions that have been made in this chapter for front-line practitioners when responding to children's concerns about adverse experiences.

---

**Box 9.1** Summary of first responses to children's concerns expressed to front-line practitioners

- Convey that you are willing and able to listen and respond to the child's concerns.
- Invite the child to communicate further, if he/she wishes.
- If appropriate, invite the child to say why he/she is concerned about a particular place or person.
- If appropriate, enquire how it was that the child became sore or developed a bruise.
- If appropriate, enquire about the child's unexplained behaviour or emotional condition.
- Avoid any specific or direct questions about adverse events, traumas or maltreatment.
- Avoid jumping to the conclusion that the child may have been harmed.
- Do not discourage a child from communicating any concerns.
- Do not pressurise a child who does not want to talk.
- It may be helpful to discuss your concerns, and possible approaches to the child, with a colleague or with the professional within your organisation with designated responsibility for child welfare and protection matters, if there is time to do so.
- Record any conversations as soon as possible after they have occurred, including the child's and the professional's questions or comments, and the sequence in which they occurred. Use as many of your own and the child's words as you can recall. Describe the setting and any emotions that were expressed. Keep all the rough notes you make.
- If you become concerned about the child's safety, avoid investigation or further assessment yourself. Discuss the situation with an experienced colleague or the relevant person within the organisation. Arrange for referral to designated child protection services if you are concerned that the child is suffering harm (the social services department, the NSPCC or the police).
- Otherwise, consider referral for other services, such as child support services.

---

Jones, D. P. H. (2003) *Communicating with Vulnerable Children*. London: Gaskell.

# CHAPTER 10

# Talking with children about adverse events during initial assessments

This chapter is concerned with the first assessments that specialist practitioners undertake for their various services and agencies. It concentrates on the exploration of possible adversity, while recognising that practitioners may well have other assessment objectives in the individual situation. First, however, a note about the terminology used in this chapter. For social workers and other professionals making an assessment of a child who may be suffering harm, this process translates into an *initial assessment*. However, other assessments, undertaken by a variety of other professionals, do not fall under Children Act guidance, for example those undertaken by child and adolescent mental health practitioners, children's guardians and those working with learning-disabled children. These latter assessments will be termed *first assessments* in this book, in order to distinguish them from initial assessments. Policy aspects of the initial assessment are considered first, then the research relevant to both initial and first assessments, followed by the implications for practice that flow from these considerations.

## The policy and procedural context

The term 'initial assessment' has particular meaning in the *Framework for the Assessment of Children in Need and Their Families* (Department of Health *et al*, 2000), which gives the government's guidance on assessments of children in need for social workers and other professionals. The social services department leads an 'initial assessment' once it has received a referral or new information about an open case. Not all requests for an initial assessment will lead to one being undertaken, because some result in decisions being made that no action is required. However, where there are concerns about a child's health and development being impaired without the provision of services, an initial assessment will be undertaken (Department of Health *et al*, 2000). This should be undertaken within seven working days of the referral. The aims of the initial assessment are to determine:

- whether the child is in need;
- the nature of any services required;

- whether a more detailed, core assessment is necessary or appropriate.

This initial assessment includes seeing the child and assessments of family members, as well as information gathering and liaison with other agencies. The direct work with children includes observation and talking with them in an age-appropriate manner. The *Assessment Framework* identifies five critical components to this direct work: seeing, observing, engaging, talking and activities with children (Department of Health *et al*, 2000, para. 3.42). It is recognised that social services departments may need to link with particular specialists from other agencies in order to inform specific aspects of such assessments.

Social workers who undertake initial assessments aim to understand the child's world and appreciate his/her perspective, through direct work with the child. The overall objective is to see whether the child's welfare is being compromised in any way (principally through adverse experiences or victimisation) and whether the child requires the provision of extra services to try to counteract that.

While the above arrangements apply to *initial assessments* undertaken by social workers, other professionals do *first assessments* as part of their services for referred children. These include child and adolescent mental health services and services for children with special needs, such as speech and language problems, communication difference, hearing impairment and learning disability. These assessments are not conducted under the umbrella of statutory government guidance. Nonetheless, because these assessments have similar aims, and because the focus in this chapter is on evaluating the possibility of victimisation or adverse experiences having befallen the child, the research and practice implications can be seen to apply both to social services department initial assessments and to first assessments.

This chapter concentrates on exploring the possibility of victimisation or adversity, in ways that can be incorporated into existing approaches to assessment. The following sources describe good practice for assessments, within different disciplines: child and adolescent mental health (Angold, 1994, 2002; Cox, 1994; Goodman & Scott, 1997; Graham *et al*, 1999; Morrison & Anders, 1999); learning disabilities (ABCD Consortium, 1993; JRF *et al*, 2001); and child and family social workers undertaking assessments of children in need (NSPCC/Chailey Heritage, 1998; Shemmings, 1998).

Children may be referred to educational or health services because they have emotional or behavioural problems or learning disabilities. Sometimes there are additional existing concerns at the point of referral about the child's welfare. When this occurs the relevant professional undertaking the first assessment is aware of the fact that, in addition to the educational or health-based reasons for referral, there are more general concerns about the child's welfare. If these concerns are sufficiently strong, they may lead to a referral to the local social services department, as a child in need. Other children are referred to health and education services with symptoms or groups of problems that in themselves raise the possibility that the child may have suffered victimisation. Examples include referral of children with sexual behaviour problems or children seen in hospital accident and emergency departments with self-harming presentations. In these circumstances, health and education practitioners will already be alert to the possibility of victimisation when planning their first assessments.

However, many presentations to health and educational special services come with no such clues as to the possibility of victimisation of the child (Jones, 1997, 2000b). This is not at all surprising, because it is well established that children are more likely to respond in a non-specific way to particular life events and stresses (Goodyer, 1991). Hence, among the common presentations, some children will have had adverse experiences that are an important aspect of their problems, notwithstanding the non-specific manner of presentation. For those providing specialised services this means that children's adverse experiences can be important factors in a wide range of different presentations. At the same time, not all children presenting with disturbance have experienced personal matters of concern. But if they have, it will be necessary for the service to be aware of this, so that it can be taken into account when planning interventions. It is also the duty of the service to be alert to the child's welfare needs, even though this may not be the primary objective of the service.

The situation is further complicated by knowledge deriving from the dynamics of victimisation, together with what is known about children's loyalties, especially to trusted attachment figures, and the impact of threats, admonitions and coercive practices on children's preparedness to reveal private or secret information (see Chapters 3 and 8). Children who have experienced maltreatment, especially in the context of close or intimate relationships, face very real dilemmas and pressures. This is reflected in the dilemmas for the professionals, who, on the one hand, want to help those children who are in complex predicaments such as these, while, on the other hand, being mindful of the dangers that derive from presumptive or biased enquiries (Ceci & Bruck, 1995). The task is thus difficult for both children and professionals. In offering the suggestions below, the complexity and difficulty of these situations are acknowledged.

The principal issues for practitioners are therefore:

*   How to explore the possibility of victimisation or adversity without suggestion.

- Whether to explore for these possibilities routinely.
- If so, how to do so.

## Research findings

The relevant studies on exploring children's concerns without suggestion have been discussed in Chapter 9 (pp. 95–97). They are equally relevant to initial assessments, and will be drawn upon when considering implications for practice, below. There are certain additional issues, however, with regard to initial assessment, which we consider next.

First, there is the question of whether to ask routinely about victimisation. Should assessments by professionals working in health and educational special services include, as a matter of routine, 'screening' questions about the possibility of adverse life experiences? Issues such as losses, deaths and illnesses are explored in any case in most assessments. The contentious issue is whether the possibility of victimisation should be directly asked about, too. In the field of child mental health, it has been shown that a change in a clinic's practice to introducing questions about the possibility of child sexual abuse increased the proportion of children who reported such a history from 7% before its introduction, to 31% once team members were trained to ask a few exploratory questions (Lanktree et al, 1991). We do not know from this study whether these accounts were subsequently verified. Critics might argue that introducing such questions raises the possibility for error, because children might think that they should answer the professional's enquiry in the affirmative. It is extremely unlikely, however, that one or two tentatively phrased screening questions would be likely to produce erroneous accounts of child maltreatment, in the absence of a generally hectoring or biased atmosphere (Ceci & Friedman, 2000).

Services vary as to whether children are routinely seen alone or always with family members and parents. Practice is likely to be dependent upon the child's age. Further, some services are more likely to see children who have been victimised than others; these would include services for children who have self-harmed and those for adolescents with eating disorders, where experiences of victimisation are probably more common than among other emotionally or psychologically troubled children. It is possible that general, open-ended questions to the family or individual children concerning possible exposure to harm, trauma or major distress are appropriate for children at less risk of harm, while a more probing enquiry might be appropriate in other circumstances, where the suggestion of victimisation is more likely. Not surprisingly, textbooks vary in their advice on this question. Some textbooks on child and adolescent psychiatry, for example,

Jones, D. P. H. (2003) *Communicating with Vulnerable Children*. London: Gaskell.

recommend asking all children about the possibility of victimisation, whereas others do not include this within their recommendations for good practice in first assessments.

In summary, there is little research to guide practitioners on whether routinely to ask children and young people about the possibility of victimisation. Advice given in the textbooks varies, unsurprisingly. It does seem that one or two questions posed in a non-leading and open-ended way are very unlikely to lead to erroneous accounts. Equally, more children do disclose victimisation if a service introduces simple questions about such matters in its assessment schema. It would certainly seem, therefore, that questions about victimisation can safely be part of a first assessment by health and education specialist services, particularly when the presentation suggests that victimisation is more likely to have occurred.

## Choice of question and approach

Precisely how questions regarding the possibility of victimisation should be phrased has been even less well researched. It is probable that a range of approaches is the best way forward, from one or two direct questions in some cases, to indirect approaches concerning discipline and family relationships in other cases.

The research that has been done has focused on the introductory questions that form part of investigative interviews for criminal justice purposes, rather than those that may be applicable to assessments of children's development needs. For example, Michael Lamb and colleagues (Orbach & Lamb, 2000; Orbach *et al*, 2000) have explored the benefits of specifically preparing children for an investigative interview. They found that a combination of instruction and practice enabled children, even as young as four years, to engage themselves more effectively in a subsequent investigative interview. The preparation consisted of conveying to the child that the adult was not in possession of the facts and that the child was the sole and only source of information. Therefore, the adult interviewer really needed to know from the child what, if anything, had happened. Orbach *et al* (2000) make the point that this is necessary because in most communications between adults and children the adults convey that they know more than the child and children have become very used to this situation. The rules of the investigative interview 'game', they maintain, are therefore substantially different from children's normal experiences of communications with adults. Part of this preparation involves helping children to say 'I don't know' if asked a question that they cannot answer. Lamb and colleagues include not only instruction in but also practice of this method of communicating in the preparatory stage of their interview protocol. They have demonstrated that children who are prepared in this way are better able to provide fuller spontaneous accounts later on in an investigative interview and appear to be more resistant to suggestive or leading questions.

These benefits of preparation, which focus on the child as the source of information and the adult as interested and curious rather than knowing and in charge of the information, have been replicated in further studies (Lamb *et al*, 1999). However, this research has been conducted in the setting of interviews designed to communicate with children where there is reasonable cause to think that a crime may have been committed (in the Lamb field studies) or where an event has occurred (in the replication studies). The assessments under consideration in this chapter are very different. In these, the type of concern is more general in nature and the approach will need to reflect this difference. There is no specific research on the benefits or otherwise of similar approaches in assessments of a child's needs. However, the situations are similar in two fundamental respects: the adult practitioner does not know what the child's experience is, and the child may well have vitally important information to convey. In this sense, therefore, research in the field of investigative interviewing could well be of relevance to initial and first assessments, and it is therefore drawn upon for recommendations, below.

Research with children reveals how much they value professionals who listen carefully, without trivialising or being dismissive, and who are non-judgemental, non-directive, honest and straightforward (Sharland *et al*, 1996; Shemmings, 1999).

## Process and decision making

There is relatively little systematic research on process and decision making when initial assessments are undertaken. We do not know the outcome of initial assessments and far less about how those decisions are made. We know that some initial assessments lead to professional concerns being allayed, and presumably children's too, because the child is discovered to be well adjusted and not burdened by adverse experiences. Equally some assessments reveal a child in need of help and assistance, and so lead to further work to determine what services may be required. A proportion of initial assessments reveal initial concerns about the child's safety and whether he/she is suffering significant harm. If the child is, further action will be required, including assessments of the child's safety under Section 47 of the Children Act (Department of Health *et al*, 1999, paras 5.33–5.38) or investigation to see whether a crime has been committed (Department of Health *et al*, 1999, paras 5.39–5.41). These issues are explored further in the next section. In terms of research to guide practitioners doing initial assessments, however, the evidential basis for decision making is relatively scanty.

There has been more research on the processes that follow the emergence of concerns about the child's safety, especially where investigative interviewing has occurred. There is some suggestion that practice is variable across the UK (Davies *et al*, 1995). Davies *et al* found that the numbers of joint investigative interviews (designed to gather evidence for criminal proceedings where a child was a victim or witness) was dramatically different in different parts of the country, with no evidence that these differences were related to regional variations in crime figures. The reasons appeared to be local practice and the thresholds that existed in different parts of the country for initiating investigative interviews. This variability was also found in an examination by the Social Services Inspectorate (SSI) of the practice of videotaping interviews with children within the UK (Department of Health, 1994). It may well be that subsequent practice has shown greater uniformity, because policy and central government guidance (Department of Health *et al*, 1999, 2000; Home Office *et al*, 2002) is now more specific about when a core assessment is more appropriate, when children should be referred to have an investigative interview and when, indeed, no further action is required at the present time. However, while government guidance sets out principles and broad signposts to guide local practice, there is still substantial scope for variation and it remains likely that the guidance will be interpreted differently across different geographical areas. It would seem important to continue to research this area.

If the situation is variable within social services and their relationship to the police, it is even more so when we look at other agencies and professionals. Results of research in the USA, where there is a mandatory requirement to report concerns about child maltreatment to social services, underline considerable variability in practice (National Center on Child Abuse and Neglect, 1988; Warner & Hansen, 1997). Some practitioners clearly flout the rules in a country where it is a criminal offence not to report concerns to a social services department. Thus, although government policy is clear, as is advice from professional organisations and regulatory bodies, there appears to be considerable variation in practice.

There has also been very little study of the contribution that professionals other than social workers make to assessments of concerns that reach social services. Early research stressed how little other professionals assisted social services departments (Gough *et al*, 1993). There is some suggestion that this situation has changed, subsequent to the introduction of the Children Act 1989, during the 1990s (Hallett & Birchall, 1992). However, we have no systematic study available of the contribution that different professionals make in the various situations that affect children. There are reports of specific areas of practice that illustrate the contribution health and other professionals can make to assessments of children in need (Department of Health, 1994; Howlin & Jones, 1996). It is clear from these, however, that health, education and social services agencies, together with voluntary organisations and other professionals, have much to gain from working together and pooling expertise when it comes to effecting good-quality assessments.

## Implications for practitioners

The principles guiding the professional approach to the child, or carers, remain the same as those applied to all communications with children (see Chapter 6). It remains crucial to do everything possible to derive the most accurate and complete account possible, and avoid approaches that may distort or contaminate the child's memory.

An initial assessment undertaken by social services will involve the child, even if this is merely a brief communication. It is likely to involve some discussion with the child's parents, other carers, or perhaps teacher, or a health professional who knows the child.

It can be difficult to decide whom to see, because at the point of referral it may not be clear what, if anything, the child's concerns comprise, or to what extent the child's carers may be implicated. Securing parental support for the child's situation is likely to be a very important factor in terms of supporting them through any interviewing process (Moston & Egleberg, 1992) and if maltreatment has occurred, supporting them through subsequent assessments to intervention (Jones & Ramchandani, 1999).

This is an example of an area where professional objectivity is key. An 'anti-parent' stance is likely to alienate parental, and especially maternal, support. Equally, uncritical support for the parent, without first considering the child's perspective and the nature of the expressed concerns, runs the risk of compromising the child. This can be particularly difficult where children have been implicitly or explicitly required to keep a secret and not reveal concerns to persons outside the immediate family.

The approach taken will depend on the source of concern. If the child raises concern independently, whether purposefully or not, a decision will have to be made as to whether it is appropriate to approach the child's parent, and if so how. (Specifically, this would be the adult with parental responsibility about whom no complaint has been made. This decision can be complicated by lack of knowledge initially as to the possible involvement of each of the adults with parental responsibility). Older children may well present independently and expect an initial discussion about their concerns and the consequences of revealing them, before parents are contacted. Older children can reasonably expect to have a greater say than younger ones in the way in which their concerns are responded to and the degree of confidentiality available to them. Teenagers may not wish their parents to be informed and, depending upon their level of understanding and appreciation of the full consequences of disclosure, their wishes carry increasing weight as they approach adulthood. At the other end of the age spectrum, young children are less likely to make deliberate disclosures of such matters as sexual or physical abuse (Davies & Westcott, 1998). Nonetheless, children in middle childhood, although more likely to make deliberate or semi-deliberate attempts to bring their situation to official attention, tend to feel excluded from decision making (Sharland *et al*, 1996) and report that events proceeded at a far faster pace than they expected (Wattam, 1992; Wade & Westcott, 1997).

The implication from these findings and observations is that it will be a matter for professional discussion and judgement as to who needs to be seen, in what order and where. Additionally, the child's capacity to consent will need to be considered. Whatever is decided should be recorded, together with the reasons for decisions reached.

In other situations, children present their concerns to a parent or carer, who subsequently contacts professionals. Similar issues arise, although in these cases the child or young person has already communicated concerns of sufficient gravity to lead to the referral. As soon as possible the detailed sequence of events, including the questions and answers involved together with the full context, should be obtained. However, the full detail generally will not be available, merely a patchy record. This can prove a problem when professionals attempt to evaluate the subsequent assessment. Although it can be problematic, as much detail as possible should be obtained about these initial communications.

Can professionals help reticent children to communicate concerns? Individual differences are likely to be crucial. The child's age is likely to have a major effect on subsequent assessment. Teenagers often have important social networks outside their immediate home and family. By contrast, young children are likely to be most dependent on their mother or primary carer. Hence, they may require greater preparation and more than one session in which to establish trust with an unknown professional from outside their family, if they are to communicate effectively. Disabled children are likely to expect professional adults to do things for and to them (Kennedy, 1992b; Marchant & Page, 1997) and may, therefore, require more extensive preparation to enable them to communicate their concerns freely, without adult direction or prompting. Issues of race and culture need to be considered – what are this individual child's racial attitudes and expectations? Professionals should also consider their own attitudes and orientation towards children from different cultural groups (Dutt & Phillips, 2000). For both disabled children and those from ethnic groups different from those of the practitioners involved, it is important to consider whether specialist help is necessary in order to communicate effectively. Do the assessing professionals have the necessary skills within their staff group, or will extra, more specialised help be required?

There are likely to be many opportunities in the course of an assessment by a practitioner to raise the possibility of adverse experiences. For example, assessments often include general discussion about sleeping routines and arrangements, and, with older children, issues of privacy and discussions about their living space. These provide opportunities for concerns to be expanded upon, if children wish. Similarly, discussions concerning discipline and what happens when the child is disobedient or poorly behaved often bring out accounts of excessive punishment as well as routine disciplines. Further, discussion about family structure and relationships is an integral part of specialist assessments. This allows for questions about whom the child likes to spend time with, and those with whom the child does not, and to whom the child is close and vice versa. Answers to these questions can be followed up with open-ended enquiries to explore the basis for these likes and dislikes.

In general, a useful approach is to pair positive experiences with potentially negative ones: a discussion about whom the child is close to can be followed by one about to whom the child does not feel so close; asking about 'the best thing that has happened to you' can be followed by asking about 'the worst thing that has happened to you'; talking about people 'you like being with' can be followed by talking about people 'you don't like being with'.

Box 10.1 makes suggestions for exploratory questions within first and initial assessments; these questions can be adapted for children of different ages. They are intended to supplement and extend the approaches outlined in Box 9.1. As a general principle, if questions such as these are used, it is important that, if the child responds in the affirmative, subsequent questions should consist of open-ended prompts and invitations to describe any adverse experiences in more detail. In this way the possible objections to exploratory questions are addressed, but at the same time the child is given the opportunity at least to raise experiences with the interviewer.

Sometimes concern about maltreatment arises during the course of an assessment. In these circumstances the child should not be prevented from communicating, but at the same time the professional should be careful not to adopt an investigating role – it is important to

Jones, D. P. H. (2003) *Communicating with Vulnerable Children*. London: Gaskell.

---

**Box 10.1** Exploratory questions

- Has anybody done anything to you that upset you? [Await response.] Or made you unhappy?
- Has any person hurt you? [Await answer.] Or touched you in a way that you didn't like?
- Or touched you in a sexual way, or in a way that you didn't like?

A circular, permission-giving question can be useful in some circumstances. For example, in circumstances where the possibility of victimisation or adversity is strong, yet the child appears to be reticent, a question like the following could be used:

- Some children talk about being upset or hurt in some way – has anything like this happened to you?

---

defer this to mandated agencies. Children should be allowed to finish raising whatever issues they wish to and then an opportunity found to refer on to the relevant professionals. This will need to be discussed with the child's parents, unless to do so would place the child at risk (Department of Health *et al*, 1999). Similarly, referral should be discussed with older child too, because often they will have concerns about confidentiality and the consequences of disclosure of information to social services departments or the police.

Referrals to specialists sometimes include an element of concern about possible harm. In these circumstances the parents or the child may already be concerned about the possibility. However, it is assumed here that the level of professional concern has not been sufficient to warrant or be accepted by local child protection professionals as requiring assessment by them. In other situations the problems presented by the child or young person are known to have a significant link with maltreatment or other traumatic events. Examples include the presentation of unusually sexualised behaviour in a young child, acts of deliberate self-harm or sudden changes in behaviour that have no other obvious explanation. In these circumstances exploratory questions are more clearly indicated, and indeed may need to go further than the very general invitations outlined in Box 9.1, and include the approaches outlined in Chapter 11.

On other occasions specialists assist social workers to make initial enquiries. For example, practitioners in learning disability or child and adolescent mental health services sometimes work with social workers to assess possible maltreatment in children with autism. These situations require rigorous planning and particular attention to each professional's role and responsibility.

# Summary

- 'Initial assessments' are brief assessments of children referred to social services departments with a request for services. The main aim is to determine whether the child is in need, what kind of additional help and services are necessary, and whether a more detailed, 'core assessment' should be undertaken. It includes an interview with the child, even if brief.
- Other professionals providing specialist services can, and often do, enquire about adverse experiences as part of their own 'first assessments'. The research considered here can be applied to both types of assessment.
- Should there be suspicions or allegations about child mal-treatment, strategy discussions and inter-agency action will then guide planning, in accordance with *Working Together to Safeguard Children* (Department of Health *et al*, 1999). The assessment process will then progress to establish whether the child's health and development are or will be impaired without the provision of services (under Section 17 of the Children Act) and, where there are concerns about a child's safety, to see whether the child is suffering or is likely to suffer harm (under Section 47), and whether action is required to secure the child's safety (Department of Health *et al*, 1999, paras 5.33–5.38; Department of Health *et al*, 2000).
- One aspect of an assessment, whether undertaken by social workers or health and education practitioners, can be to discover whether the child has been victimised or has concerns about adverse experiences, and if so what the child's perspective is on this. These enquiries are part of a broader assessment. For social workers this will comprise an initial assessment that is aimed at understanding the child's world, while at the same time the interviewer remains alert to any concerns about adverse experiences. Health and educational specialist services have their own established practices for undertaking 'first assessments'; however, when appropriate they too can adopt the approach to exploring the possibility of victimisation described in this chapter.
- In all initial and first assessments, the practitioner's style is very important. Professionals need to convey a willingness to listen and respond to any experiences that a child wishes to convey. They should also demonstrate an interest in the child's perspective and convey that they are not in possession of the facts – in this instance it is the child who is.
- Practitioners can employ questions that are effective in inviting children to recount experiences of adversity while at the same time avoiding inappropriate suggestion and undue influence.

  Jones, D. P. H. (2003) *Communicating with Vulnerable Children*. London: Gaskell.

- Exploratory enquiry often yields valuable information about adverse events that children have experienced. If limited to one or two questions, and framed in an exploratory and tentative way, it is unlikely to lead to a false or spurious account.

- If a child does describe adverse or traumatic events, it is important that the practitioner does not stop or divert a child who is freely describing such experiences. On the other hand, it may be inappropriate to invite the child to elaborate any further, particularly if it seems as though a crime may have been committed, of which the child is the victim or witness. In these instances referral to the appropriate statutory authorities is the appropriate next step, as set out in *Working Together to Safeguard Children* (Department of Health *et al*, 1999).

- Exploratory approaches are not confined to questions alone, but importantly involve a range of opportunities that enable a child to express any concerns. These indirect approaches include talking about family relationships, discipline, the child's likes and dislikes, and so on.

- At the end of an initial or first assessment the practitioner should prepare the child for any further assessments considered necessary. This would include information about what might happen next, and whom the child might meet. Future possibilities include: no further action; the provision of services and review after a period of time; progression to a core assessment, which would include a more in-depth session or sessions with the child; or, in situations involving the possibility of crime, an investigative interview under the auspices of *Achieving Best Evidence* (Home Office *et al*, 2002).

- In those cases where an investigative interview has already occurred, but criminal proceedings are not being pursued, and in the other cases of broader-based concerns about the child's welfare, assessments of the type described in this chapter are appropriate.

- Whatever the outcome of the initial or first assessment, a full record should be made of what both child and practitioner have said. It should include the full sequence and context of the communication, together with observations made concerning the child's non-verbal communication and activities or play during the assessment.

# CHAPTER 11

# In-depth interviews with children

The policy context for in-depth interviews is considered first in this chapter. Next, the research and its practice implications are reviewed. After the evidence has been considered, a suggested schema for undertaking such interviews is set out. This last section contains detailed recommendations for talking with children during in-depth interviews.

## The policy and procedural context

Communicating with children is an essential part of assessments undertaken by social workers and others who work with children and families. *Core assessments* are defined as in-depth assessments that address the central or most important aspects of the needs of the child and the capacity of the parents or carers to respond to these needs (Department of Health *et al*, 2000, para. 3.11). These assessments draw upon a series of direct and indirect sources of information, including the child, family, school and health workers (Department of Health *et al*, 2000, para. 3.39). The child component of the core assessment is wide ranging and includes, through direct work with the child, shared activities, interviews, questionnaires and play that is age and culturally appropriate (Department of Health *et al*, 2000, para. 3.39). The process is led by social services, but it almost always involves other agencies and professionals (Department of Health *et al*, 2000, para. 3.11).

There is a requirement for the identification of significant harm and the protection of children from it. Hence the emphasis of the government's guidance is on the necessity of communication with children, both when needs in general are being assessed (Department of Health *et al*, 2000, chapter 3, especially paras 3.20, 3.21, 3.37–3.45) and in the specific instance of establishing whether there is reasonable cause to suspect that the child is suffering significant harm (Section 47 enquiries; see Department of Health *et al*, 1999, especially para. 5.36). It is important to stress that 'assessment of what is happening to a child in these circumstances (where harm is suspected or alleged) is not a separate or different activity but continues the same process, although the pace and scope of assessment may well have changed' (Department of Health *et al*, 2000, para. 3.15).

As already stated, where there are concerns about the child suffering possible harm, the guidance in *Working Together to Safeguard Children*

Jones, D. P. H. (2003) *Communicating with Vulnerable Children*. London: Gaskell.

(Department of Health *et al*, 1999, paras 5.33–5.38) applies. Further, in those cases where a crime is thought to have been committed, the guidance on investigative interviewing is set out in *Achieving Best Evidence* (Home Office *et al*, 2002).

In this chapter we consider what evidence there is to guide practitioners and the implications from best practice for direct work and interviews with children when an investigative interview is not considered to be appropriate, yet an assessment of the child is required. Not only is direct work with children essential to understanding their needs and the situation in which they find themselves, but it is also necessary if we are to address their right to be involved and consulted about matters that affect them (Department of Health *et al*, 2000).

A core assessment interview with the child is likely to be a wide-ranging enquiry about the needs of that child. In this chapter we concentrate only on that component of such an assessment that is concerned with exploring the child's experiences of any adversity: it is recognised that direct work with the child as part of a core assessment will be wider in scope than the approach set out here.

---

**Box 11.1** Occasions when professionals other than social workers undertake in-depth interviews

- When significant adversity or possible maltreatment is unexpectedly presented during assessment.
- When adversity or possible maltreatment emerges in response to an open-ended enquiry or initial assessment (see Chapters 9 and 10).
- When they are requested to undertake an assessment by social services before the start of family proceedings (see note below).
- When they are requested to undertake an assessment during family proceedings (Department of Health *et al*, 2000, paras 3.20–3.27 and appendix D).

'Family proceedings' is a term that is defined statutorily in Section 8 of the Children Act 1989. It includes all public law applications (care, adoption, emergency protection, contact) and a range of private law matters, principally centring on divorce and separation, including applications under Section 8 for contact, residence, specific issue and prohibited steps orders. Assessments can occur before family court proceedings have begun, either because they are not at that time anticipated, or because they are requested in order to contribute to an assessment and inform subsequent decision making on behalf of the child (Department of Health *et al*, 2000, paras 3.20, 3.21, 3.26). Once a child is subject to a family proceedings court application, the leave of the court is required before a child is medically or psychiatrically examined for the preparation of expert evidence in subsequent proceedings. In practice, the scope of any proposed assessment will be discussed with legal advisers. Emergency assessment and intervention, of course, are not subject to this requirement, when delay may harm the child (Department of Health *et al*, 2000, paras 3.28–3.30).

---

What follows is orientated towards the requirements of social workers undertaking interviews with children within the government's assessment framework (Department of Health *et al*, 2000). However, as indicated, there are numerous implications for the work of other professionals who, while undertaking their own specialist activities, also communicate with a child about possible adversity as part of their assessment work (e.g. child and adolescent mental health practitioners and those working with children with learning disabilities or communication impairments). Sometimes this work occurs before any social work involvement or the start of family proceedings. At other times professionals other than social workers communicate with a child in a planned way. This is because children respond non-specifically to discrete stressors, such as witnessing violence or being maltreated (Chapter 4) and hence, unless a history of victimisation is known about before referral, practitioners may find themselves assessing what appears to be a straightforward problem, only to discover significant adversity unfolding during the course of the assessment. Box 11.1 lists the planned and unplanned occasions for professionals other than social workers who might undertake an in-depth interview, either in whole or in part. We return below to the strategic planning implications that arise for such professionals, which have been set out in order to ensure they work within the guidelines established by the government in *Working Together to Safeguard Children* (Department of Health *et al*, 1999).

## Research findings and practice implications

Practitioners are faced with a series of key questions when undertaking in-depth interviews. In the following sub-sections we consider the principal issues, listed in the Box 11.2, by examining research evidence, before reviewing the practice implications that follow from these. After these issues have been considered, an overview of the main practice

---

**Box 11.2** Principal issues for practitioners undertaking in-depth interviews

- What are the most useful approaches for obtaining accurate and useful accounts of adverse experiences from children (including the length of interviews and whether parents should be present)?
- To what extent should interviews be planned in advance, and if so, how?
- Should children be prepared for interviews of this kind, if so how?
- What should happen in the introductory or rapport phase of an interview?
- What is the place for indirect, creative approaches to interviewing children?
- Should in-depth interviews have a set structure? If so, what should that comprise?
- How should in-depth interviews be recorded?

---

Jones, D. P. H. (2003) *Communicating with Vulnerable Children*. London: Gaskell.

implications is set out, followed by a recommended schema for undertaking in-depth interviews, which is based on the available research and consensus statements.

## Obtaining accurate and useful accounts

### Research findings

It is self-evident that an accurate and reliable account is required from children if their needs are to be identified. Needs assessment informs subsequent decision making, from the perspective of both child welfare and family or criminal justice. The effect of error are serious and a mistake can cause major harm in itself to the child and others. As we have seen in Chapter 3, the consequences of error is as important in civil and family proceedings as they are in criminal proceedings. It is therefore critically important that practitioners use the most reliable approaches for obtaining information when they interview children. There has been a great deal of research, conducted in both laboratories and the real world of practice (e. g. Davey & Hill, 1999) that can help practitioners decide which approaches produce the most reliable accounts by children. A number of up-to-date reviews of this work are available (Ceci & Bruck, 1995; Poole & Lamb, 1998; Westcott *et al*, 2002; Westcott & Jones, 2003). The research base for the best methods of obtaining accurate accounts have been discussed in previous chapters (see Chapters 2 and 6, in particular). Some of the key findings are listed in Box 11.3. We will also consider other issues that may affect accuracy, such as how long should sessions last and is accuracy affected by having the child's parents or other carer present?

### How long should sessions last?

There are some issues about which there is little or no systematic research – examples include how long interviews should last, and the benefits or otherwise of having a parent or support person present for the child during in-depth interviews. Instead, we need to consider alternative sources of information to inform these decisions. For example, key factors with regard to the duration of an interview would seem to be the child's attention span and capacity to concentrate on the task in hand, the interviewer's awareness of the child's condition and the interviewer's response to this. Indeed, many of the core skills outlined in Chapter 6 are relevant in this regard (especially practitioners' respect for the individual child, their capacity to manage and contain the assessment, and their awareness of the overall transaction).

### Should a parent be present?

The value of having a parent or other supportive adult present in an in-depth interview raises important dilemmas. On the one hand, research

**Box 11.3** Summary of the principal findings relating to the accuracy of children's accounts of adverse events

- Children produce highly accurate, although typically brief, accounts concerning adverse events, in response to open, general invitations.
- The responses of young and learning-disabled children are likely to be especially brief.
- Subsequent questions may, but do not necessarily, lead to inaccuracy. Accuracy is preserved if the interviewer is free from bias, does not use suggestion and does not lead the child to a predetermined answer.
- Some types of questions are more suggestive than others.
- The most accurate questions are open, general invitations or non-directive questions.
- Errors become increasingly likely to occur when questions become more option-posing in nature (also known as closed or forced choice) and especially when they are suggestive, leading or misleading.
- Suggestible interviewing involves imparting the interviewer's agenda upon the child. When this occurs the child's original memory becomes overwritten, supplemented or coexists with the newly implanted idea.
- Children are more suggestible if the interviewer repeatedly makes false suggestions, creates a stereotype about a person, asks the child repeatedly to visualise a false event, when the child is asked about things that happened a long time ago, or if the interviewer uses anatomically detailed dolls. These effects are made worse if interviewers are biased, pursuing their own agenda and are over-authoritative in manner.
- More than one session or interview may enable the child to describe further information, especially if adverse events have been experienced repeatedly. In these circumstances particular care is required to keep the questioning free from suggestion.
- If children are questioned with general, open-ended questions, then repeated interviews are likely to be highly accurate. However, if the questions are more suggestive or leading, then accuracy declines sharply.
- Asking the same question repeatedly within one interview may lead to error, particularly if the questions are direct or leading in nature.
- Children who have experienced similar adverse events on numerous occasions may have difficulty describing these in a single interview session, and therefore often require more than one session and special skills in order to help them delineate discrete events. Conversely, unskilful questioning poses special difficulties for children who have experienced events repeatedly.
- Children, like adults, do lie and otherwise deceive, as well as becoming confused or misled by interviewers' practice.

studies emphasise the importance of social support for children in these circumstances. Conversely, the parent may influence the child, knowingly or otherwise, and this could lead the child to make errors or to omit sensitive material. Additionally, the practitioner may not know at the outset the extent to which any particular adult may be directly or indirectly involved in any adverse experiences the child wants to communicate.

It may be possible to involve the child in deciding whether to include a particular adult. Involving the child in decision making is known to be of benefit, generally. However, this too can be complicated if the child's relationship with the adult is compromised or otherwise affected by the very adversity that is being assessed (Tan & Jones, 2001). Examples include children whose security of attachment has been affected by abuse and violence, such that they may find autonomous thinking and communicating difficult, if not impossible (Jones *et al*, 1994; Dickenson & Jones, 1995).

## Implications for practitioners

The elements of successful communication have been summarised in Chapter 6. It has been found that some degree of structure to the interview helps to lower the frequency of leading and other suggestive questioning, and raises the frequency of the more accurate questioning techniques, at least in the field of investigative interviewing for criminal purposes (Lamb *et al*, 1999). Although equivalent studies have not been done for in-depth interviews in the family justice arena, both case-based accounts, such as those of the Cleveland enquiry (Butler-Sloss, 1998) and Orkney enquiry (Clyde, 1992), and clinical experience (Ceci

---

**Box 11.4** Obtaining reliable accounts

*Approaches to be encouraged*
- The use of approaches and questions that invite free report from the child.
- The use of specific questions where necessary to establish details and, where used, preferably pairing them with subsequent open-ended questions and invitations.
- The maintenance of neutrality but not indifference towards the child.
- Knowledge of the circumstances in which children are vulnerable to suggestion.
- The maintenance of an open mind and the avoidance of personal biases and any presumptions held about the child's experiences.

*Approaches to avoid*
- The obtaining of 'disclosures' at the expense of reliable accounts.
- The use of leading and suggestive questions.
- Coercion or pressure on the child to go in a particular direction or another.
- The use of the practitioner's authority over the child and the imparting of expectations, impressions or pressure to respond in a particular way.
- The conveying of bias or presupposition, or the maintenance of a personal agenda during interviews with a child.
- Repeated questions about one issue during a single interview.

---

& Bruck, 1995; Horowitz *et al*, 1995) suggest that the picture is similar. Based on these findings, the practice implications for practitioners seeking to obtain reliable accounts are summarised in Box 11.4, in which approaches to avoid are distinguished from those to be encouraged.

## Advance planning

### Research findings

Planning is important for a number of reasons, not least to ensure that the assessment is as fruitful as possible. It allows practitioners to find the least disruptive or distressing way of approaching and interviewing the child, and reduces the potential for repetition or duplication by different professionals and agencies (Department of Health *et al*, 2000, para. 3.37). This crucial area of practice shapes the future process and the outcome of cases (Adcock, 2001). However, the planning process itself has been little studied, although it can be said that the results of lack of planning have emerged from qualitative and process research of the child welfare system (Department of Health, 1995) and case-based studies. Problems have included: unresolved differences between professionals, resulting in biased work and compromised outcomes for children; rushed assessments; alienation of parents and children; lack of partnership working with parents and children; and problems for professionals identifying different roles and multiple responsibilities in relation to child welfare, protection and criminal justice. The government's policy and procedural guidelines, especially those of the past decade, have in the main been designed to overcome these shortcomings, as well as being directed towards obtaining the best outcomes for children.

One outcome of planning may be a decision to have a preparatory session with the child. This is considered further, below. First, however, it should be pointed out that so-called 'blind' interviews have been recommended or proposed by some authors, principally on the grounds that they prevent prejudgement and bias on the part of the interviewer, who may otherwise be tempted merely to confirm an existing view during the interview with the child (see Chapter 6; also Cantlon *et al*, 1996; Jones, 1996; Poole & Lamb, 1998, pp. 112–114). In these, no prior information is available to the interviewer, except the name and age of the child. However, there have been no studies of the quality of information obtained in blind interviews, even though it can be demonstrated that blind interviews can be productive, at least with older children.

Poole & Lamb (1998) discuss the disadvantages of blind interviewing. They point to the difficulties of obtaining rapport when there is no information about the child's personal or family history, and the problems of introducing the topic of abuse if there is no information as to how the complaint arose. They also suggest that blind interviewing may, in fact, result in less consideration of alternative hypotheses. Because in-depth interviews generally have a broader remit than investigation of the possibility of criminal activities, the arguments against so-called blind interviewing are even more compelling, and the approach is less likely to be helpful. However, the approach has underlined the importance of containing pre-existing bias and so, to this extent at least, the research is relevant here.

## Implications for practitioners

Although there is little research to draw upon, it is clear that establishing the purpose of assessing a particular child is a bedrock for good practice. Planning should allow the practitioner to determine the main purpose and any specific objectives of the assessment, and to identify particular issues to do with an individual child and family relevant to obtaining a good outcome from the session. In addition to the general overall aim of identifying the needs of the child, various specific objectives may be identified, too, for example:

- To address the rights of the child and obtain information to guide decisions involving consent and confidentiality (Department of Health *et al*, 2000, paras 3.46– 3.57; Department of Health, 2001; Tan & Jones, 2001).
- To understand the child's views, wishes, feelings and attitudes about, for example, particular persons, situations or contact arrangements.
- To assess the child's psychological condition.
- To make an assessment of the child's developmental status.
- To determine whether the child should be told particular information about which he/she is not yet aware, such as that concerning disease or illness of the child or in a parent, or information concerning birth origins, perhaps as recently revealed through DNA testing.
- To explore possible adverse experiences, especially where a decision has already been made not to proceed to a joint investigation, following the guidance outlined for gathering evidence for prospective criminal proceedings (Department of Health *et al*, 1999; Home Office *et al*, 2002).
- To assess whether the child may have harmed others or become involved with other children in activities where being victimised appears to have overlapped with victimising others (in more clear-cut situations where the child is thought to have directly harmed others, then the arrangements outlined in *Achieving Best Evidence*, para 2.151, apply; Home Office *et al*, 2002).

**Box 11.5** Items to consider when planning an in-depth interview

*A review of existing information.*
- What information is already available?
- Is a detailed sequence of the evolution of concerns available, and if not, can it be obtained?
- What new information is required and what can be obtained through communicating with the child directly?
- What is known about the child's developmental status, language, ethnicity, culture and progress at school?
- What is known about the child's friendships and family relationships?
- What is known about the child's and parents' wishes and views?

*Aims and objectives*
- What is the main purpose of the interview and are there any subsidiary aims?
- Are there any other alternative possibilities or explanations that may need to be explored during the interview?

*Children's and parents' rights*
- What are the issues in relation to consent of the child and parent(s)?
- Are there issues with regard to confidentiality that can be anticipated?

*Whom to interview*
- Which child or children will be seen and in what order, especially with respect to siblings and other family members?

*Who will undertake the assessment?*
- Are there any special needs with respect to communication, language or culture? If so, are staff with particular expertise required?

*Approach and introduction*
- How is the child going to be approached, and if necessary prepared for an interview?
- Who will do the introductions?
- How will the child be transported (if applicable)?

*Collecting information*
- What methods for collecting information will be used? Are any question-naires or scales likely to be used to supplement an interview?

*Site for the interview*
- Where will the assessment take place?
- Is it appropriate to see the child at home, or in some other setting?

*Resources*
- Are particular resources required in terms of the age of the child (e.g. appropriateness of setting for young children and teenagers)?
- Are any special resources required for addressing special needs, impairments or disabilities?

*What time-scale is anticipated?*
- Allow time for settling in, obtaining consent, debriefing and feeding back after any session, and making arrangements for subsequent actions.

*Analysis*
- How will the interview be analysed?
- Who will be involved in doing this and how will the results or outcome be fed back to child, family and other professionals?

*Recording*
- How will the interview be recorded?
- Who will have access to this record and where will it be stored?
- Will it be able to be copied for use by other practitioners?

Jones, D. P. H. (2003) *Communicating with Vulnerable Children*. London: Gaskell.

The principal components of a plan for an assessment have been listed in the government's assessment framework (Department of Health *et al*, 2000, paras 3.37–3.40.). Box 11.5 summarises the main areas to be considered when planning an in-depth interview. Most of the items listed have been derived from the assessment framework, but may also be derived from the above discussion.

## Preparation of the child

### Research findings

Very little is known from field-based research studies about what happens in typical cases during any preparation period, or what influence the management of this interim period has on children's subsequent accounts. However, extrapolating from the concerns about children's suggestibility (see Chapter 2) it would certainly be wise to pay attention to what happens at this time, in order to prevent untoward negative effects on children and their memory of events. Younger children and those with learning disabilities may be especially prone to being influenced by the perceived expectations of the adults who are providing care for them.

It has been demonstrated that preparation helps to produce more accurate and complete accounts from children (Saywitz & Snyder, 1993). Nonetheless, there may be pressure on practitioners to proceed as quickly as possible with an assessment interview, as parents will ask questions and want to know about any possible harm that their child has suffered. Children are likely to be affected by their parents' disturbance or distress. In a study of children's and parents' reaction to sexual abuse investigations, the parents' state of personal distress at discovering that their child might have been maltreated was often not fully taken into account by professionals (Sharland *et al*, 1996). It is important to remember that a common message from a child's perspective is that professionals proceed too quickly and the child does not feel involved in what is happening (Wade & Westcott, 1997) – and parents feel similarly (Sharland *et al*, 1996).

### Implications for practitioners

On the one hand, an immediate interview prevents the child being subjected to improper influences or pressures from parents or others. On the other hand, time spent preparing the child for any substantive interview can be very valuable. Equally, preparation of the child means that the planning of the interview and any parallel assessments of the child, any other children and family members is afforded more time for proper consideration. Box 11.6 sets out the areas that can benefit from preparing children for interview. Sometimes, an extended period of time will be needed in order to adequately prepare a child for an assessment

---

**Box 11.6** Possible areas to cover with the child in preparation for an in-depth interview

- Familiarisation of child and interviewer.
- Identification of the child's views, feelings and concerns.
- Opportunity to involve the child in the process of assessment.
- Explanation of the purpose of the forthcoming interview.
- Assessment of consent (or at least, less formally, assent) to the interview process.
- Discussion about confidentiality concerns.
- Discussion and evaluation of the role and presence of parents, or other support persons.
- Outline developmental assessment and identification of any special communication requirements.
- Introduction to, and initial trial of, the principles of the interview (e.g. the child as the expert, the need for free narrative and the child saying as much as possible about the events recalled).

---

interview. Examples include when children are reluctant to communicate (yet professional concern is high), where they may have serious mental health problems, or major disability, and sometimes where children are very young. Extended preparation may be needed in order to allay, or address, excessive fearfulness, or to fully assess special needs or circumstances, or to respond to an older child's concerns about confidentiality and the consequences of disclosing their experiences.

Parents and carers require preparation too. This is considered further in Chapter 13. Overall, the arguments for preparation outweigh those against it, except in situations where it is considered that the child will face inordinately severe pressure unless an assessment is undertaken swiftly and without any further preparation. Even in these circumstances, some preparation time is necessary, even though it may have to be undertaken within one brief meeting with the child.

## The introductory or rapport phase of the interview

### Research findings

The majority of our understanding in this area comes from field studies of interviews with children conducted for criminal purposes, rather than in connection with civil proceedings. However, some of the same problems during this introductory phase have been observed in interviews conducted for family justice purposes (Butler-Sloss, 1988; Clyde, 1992; Ceci & Bruck, 1995) and to this extent the findings from criminal investigations can be helpful and are therefore considered in some detail.

Jones, D. P. H. (2003) *Communicating with Vulnerable Children*. London: Gaskell.

A study of video-taped interviews undertaken for criminal investigations in the UK (Davies *et al*, 1995) concluded that there was normally a rapport stage to the interview, but the ground rules of the interview were frequently omitted. The authors found that, in general, an acceptable degree of rapport between interviewer and child was established. However, in a quarter of all cases the alleged offence was mentioned during this phase, that is, before the attempt to elicit a free narrative account.

Warren *et al* (1996) found that in most interviews a degree of rapport was established but that the interview was nonetheless mostly led by the adult, who also primarily used specific rather than open-ended questions and talked much more than the child. Other commentators have criticised child interviewers for mechanical rapport building. In these studies, brief stereotyped direct questions were put to children in order to build rapport, and interviewers' responses were seemingly lukewarm, as though 'interviewers seemed to regard rapport building as a formality that must be observed, before getting down to the real business of talking about abuse' (Wood *et al*, 1996). Wood *et al* were also concerned about overly formal, apparently unconcerned, non-verbal behaviour by interviewers, as well as excessive use of closed questions early in the interview. They were particularly critical of children being asked a string of questions about age, birthday, name of school, colours and the difference between truth and lies early in interviews, as this is likely to lead to either a sense of failure in younger children or boredom and restlessness in the older ones. These negative findings have been stressed here because they illustrate some of the problems with this stage as it is sometimes practised in both the UK and the USA.

Some practitioners express the view that this stage is not very helpful, particularly if they have had preliminary discussions or contact with the child and feel they have already established rapport. They nonetheless feel compelled to proceed with rapport building, because the guidance on interviewing for criminal justice purposes states that this should occur. However, it is known that children are more likely to convey information in an interview if they feel they understand its purpose, are reasonably at ease, and feel supported both by the interviewer and by the context in which the session occurs. Retrospectively, children who have been through investigative interviews often do not report this, and to the contrary feel confused, rushed and under pressure (Ceci & Bruck, 1995; Westcott & Davis, 1996). It seems, also, that children need to establish the limits of confidentiality, particularly with respect to video-recording and whether a parent or carer will be viewing their interview (either by watching a tape later on, or by being present, or by remotely viewing the session via a monitor).

It has been established that the way in which the initial introduction is conducted has a significant effect on the subsequent ability of the child freely to recall information about issues of possible concern in the main part of the interview (Sternberg *et al*, 1997) and improves children's ability to respond to misleading questions (Gee *et al*, 1999). It appears that the best way of conveying the ground rules is through children practising recalling a neutral event at the interviewer's request (Orbach *et al*, 2000).

Warren *et al* (1996) list the assumptions that children are likely to make, and which therefore need to be countered by the interviewer during this introductory phase. They are as follows:

- Every question must be answered even if it is not understood.
- Every question has a right or wrong answer.
- The interviewer already knows what happened and that, if the child is in doubt, the interviewer is the one who is correct.
- The child is not allowed to answer 'I don't know', or to ask for clarification.

It is plain from this list that simply suggesting to children that they can say 'I don't know' is unlikely to be sufficient as a ground rule instruction to counter all the presumptions that the child is likely to bring to the interview. If the influence of perceived authority and the context of anxiety, stress and concern about the future consequences of disclosure are added to this, it is easy to see how error can be introduced. By contrast, the opportunities for preventing error become clearer.

Explaining the ground rules to children reduces the number of subsequent inaccuracies in the accounts of events offered even by young children (Mulder & Vrij, 1996), especially if the interviewer introduces leading suggestions about maltreatment. However, instructing children to say they 'don't know' may lead to some children using this as a let-out clause when faced with difficult or embarrassing memories in the subsequent interview. Hence, the ground rules need to be set out, but also be backed up with a practice session, dealing with a neutral subject. The neutral subject could consist of a recent outing, trip or holiday.

## Implications for practitioners

The introductory phase is important. It establishes the tone of the interview that is to follow. It allows for the ground rules to be stated and tested out on neutral subject matter. The ethos of the in-depth interview is different from other conversations with children: in the former, the child is the expert and knows more about the focus of concern than the interviewer. Therefore, in the introductory phase, the child should learn to contradict the interviewer if necessary.

This phase also allows particular issues to be explored if they have not already been covered, for example confidentiality, consent and the child's level of understanding. It allows for a degree of reciprocal

Jones, D. P. H. (2003) *Communicating with Vulnerable Children*. London: Gaskell.

warmth and mutual understanding to be established between child and interviewer, which is essential for any successful interview.

A good introduction and rapport phase is insurance, to the extent that it increases the child's ability to reject any erroneous suggestions inadvertently introduced by the practitioner later on. Its duration needs to take into account the extent of any preparation that has already taken place.

## The place of indirect, creative approaches to interviewing children

This question is explored more fully in the next chapter. However, various props, drawings and other techniques designed to help children communicate more freely have long been used and found to be of value in work with children therapeutically and in educational settings. These tools can be extremely helpful in the context of in-depth interviews, provided they are not linked to leading and suggestive questioning processes. If they are, inaccuracy can result and hence such techniques should be used with care. Overall, such techniques should be best regarded as a non-verbal equivalent of direct and focused questioning styles, in terms of their effect on accuracy. We will return to this topic in more detail in Chapter 12.

## The structure of in-depth interviews

### Research findings

Reliable accounts are key to successful and fair decisions in the field of children's welfare. Reliable accounts demand accurate ways of interviewing and questioning children about possible adverse events. Researchers (e.g. Lamb *et al*, 1998) and case analyses (Butler-Sloss, 1988; Clyde, 1992; Ceci & Bruck, 1995; *Re H*, 2000) emphasise that practitioners within the family justice system do not always employ accurate methods. Should interviewers therefore adopt the same structured approach advocated by Lamb *et al* (1998) for criminal purposes? These studies have demonstrated the benefits of a structured approach to questioning, as a means of obtaining more and better information from children in criminal investigations.

### Implications for practitioners

It is probable that the children's situations are too diverse and uncertain for a wholly structured approach to be applied within the child welfare field. The assessments undertaken are likely to cover much wider ground and are not solely focused on recalled events of the kind that might concern the criminal justice system. However, some of the main features of a structured approach can be usefully imported, especially those designed to encourage initial, open-ended, introductory questions, and the methods outlined for moving from a rapport-gaining stage to a focus on events of concern. Some degree of structure is therefore preferable for in-depth interviews in order to avoid the pitfalls of leading and suggestive questioning.

In the absence of clear-cut research findings, it seems reasonable to adopt a simple schema that can be applied to the variety of circumstances encountered within the field of welfare assessments, which preserves the emphasis on open-ended enquiry, while avoiding leading and suggestive practices. Such a schema is set out in the last part of this chapter.

## Recording interviews

In-depth interviews require adequate preparation and should be accurately recorded, because of both their significance in terms of planning for the child's future and the contribution the findings may make to subsequent legal proceedings, principally in the family court.

In experimental situations, video-recording does not appear to reduce the accuracy of children's accounts (Endres *et al*, 1999). However, practitioners observe that children are sometimes very sensitive to video-taping and may ask 'Will I be on telly?' or occasionally show particular concern when video-taping has been a component of their adverse experience. One problem is that this might not always be known in advance (because if it is suspected it is likely the child would already have been diverted for an investigative interview). Hopefully this issue will have been raised with the child in preparation for an interview, but sometimes either this phase has not occurred or it suddenly becomes especially poignant for the child when faced with a video-camera.

It has been established that children benefit from being involved in decisions about activities that affect them. This principle can be applied to which form of recording is the most appropriate.

### Implications for practitioners

The practitioner will need to balance the needs and wishes of the child with those of the system, which requires information for decision making. Sometimes this creates conflicts. For example, the family justice system prefers a video-taped interview to be available. However, this may not be possible, either because of child factors, or because the child's disclosures in an in-depth interview were not initially anticipated. Hence, in practice the essential issue is to have a good-quality, accurate record. The alternatives to video-taping are audio-recording (modern audio equipment renders this option a useful compromise solution) or making a contemporaneous record through detailed note taking, supplemented by details added from memory immediately after

Jones, D. P. H. (2003) *Communicating with Vulnerable Children*. London: Gaskell.

the session. If audio-taping is chosen, it will still need to be complemented with contemporaneous notes, especially concerning the child's activity level, demeanour and interaction with the interviewer. It is essential to keep any rough notes that are made, even if these are subsequently superseded by more detailed notes, because the original jottings can provide invaluable evidence in legal proceedings, whether family or criminal justice ones.

---

**Box 11.7** Summary of the principal implications from research for practitioners undertaking in-depth interviews

- A child's free account is preferable to answers obtained from specific questions, because it is likely to be fuller and more accurate.
- If direct questions are used, they should not be leading in type, repeated frequently during the interview, or associated with any other type of pressure from the professional. They should be followed by open-ended questions, or invitations to the child to say more.
- Practitioners should avoid bias and presupposition.
- Interviews should normally be planned in advance. This enables clear identification of the purpose of the interview.
- It is useful to prepare children for in-depth interviews, so that they know what to expect and in order to involve them in the process.
- In-depth interviews should normally have an introductory, rapport-building phase.
- A flexibly employed structure to the session is useful.
- Interviews should be recorded carefully in the most appropriate way for the individual circumstances.
- The practitioner should remember that false or erroneous accounts can emanate from children, adult carers or from professional practice.
- Any interviews with children should be based on established principles of professional good practice (see Chapter 6).
- It is essential to listen to and understand the child.
- It is essential to convey genuine empathic concern.
- It is essential to convey the view that it is the child who is the expert, not the professional.
- It is easier for practitioners to develop and maintain the qualities and competencies outlined above if they work within an environment that encourages critical review of practice, if they seek frequent updates on research findings and consensus statements, and if they have opportunities for continuing professional development.
- When practitioners are undertaking assessments, including in-depth interviews, they should be aware of the relevant law and guidance, including *Working Together to Safeguard Children* (Department of Health *et al*, 1999). This advice applies to all practitioners who work with children and not just to social workers. These responsibilities involve reporting the outcome of assessments to any other agency or group of professionals, as appropriate, including the provision of reports if necessary, and giving evidence to the family justice courts.

---

## Summary of practice implications for in-depth interviews

The principal implications for practitioners derived from the relevant research are listed in Box 11.7 in note form. There is some repetition so that this list can act as an aide memoire for busy practitioners.

# A schema for undertaking in-depth interviews

How can the implications and approaches summarised above and drawn from research and practice be applied in the field?

The need for planning and preparation has already been stressed. One or more preparatory sessions may well have occurred before a substantive session is conducted. At the least, introductions will be necessary and the relevant issues concerning consent addressed. We have already noted that sometimes the need for an in-depth interview was not apparent in advance. In these circumstances, some of the issues considered above in relation to preparing a child for interview will need to be covered during the introductory part of the interview (see below). Whatever the situation, a format for these interviews is presented below. It should be reiterated that many such interviews constitute only one part of a social worker's direct work with a child as part of a core assessment (Department of Health *et al*, 2000). Other professionals (e.g. health professionals), in circumstances such as those outlined in Box 11.1, however, conduct some interviews. The approach recommended here comprises the following phases:

- Introductory, rapport-gaining phase.
- Enquiry into suspected adverse experiences.
- Further exploration.
- Closure.

It is envisaged that this schema will be useful as an outline skeleton and will require adaptation to individual circumstances.

## Introductory, rapport-gaining phase

The main aims of this phase of the interview are:

- to establish a working relationship with the child;
- to engage the child's interest in the session;
- to place the child or young person at ease.

If a preparatory session has not occurred previously, it would be necessary to deal with some of these items in this phase of the main interview. Even if there has been a successful preparatory session, the interviewer can use this phase of the interview to talk about a neutral matter in order to practise the ground rules of the interview that will

Jones, D. P. H. (2003) *Communicating with Vulnerable Children*. London: Gaskell.

follow. That is, the central ethos of an in-depth interview is that the child is the expert, whereas the adult is not. Hence, to choose a neutral subject, which the child has knowledge of but the interviewer does not, provides an excellent opportunity for practising the style of the session that will be required later on. Possible approaches might be to discover how the child travelled to the interview, or any particular interests the child has or activities the child has taken part in recently.

The interviewer establishes the relationship with the child by talking about general aspects of the child's life, such as school or friendships. It may not be appropriate to talk about home life, particularly if the child's concerns centre on this area of life: at this early stage the interviewer generally avoids the specific areas of concern that have led to the in-depth interview. Some children and young people will not appreciate this. For example, some adolescents may find the inter- viewer's avoidance of what they know to be the subject of concern irritatingly patronising. However, provided the interviewer is aware of the nature of the interaction, this can be spotted early and responded to flexibly.

It may be necessary for practitioners to explain who they are, if this has not been done at a preparatory stage. Such introductions should be brief and avoid specific reference to matters of concern. It is perhaps best for practitioners to avoid identifying themselves as someone who protects children or ensures they are safe because this establishes a particular agenda for the session. Equally, it would be inappropriate for the practitioner to educate the child about correct words for parts of the body, or personal safety issues, or to pass an opinion on what adults should or should not do. The aim of in-depth interviews is to make an assessment of the child from a number of perspectives and, with regard to safety issues, to find out what, if anything, may have happened, and if something has, to discover as much detail as possible about it.

Once rapport has been established, the interviewer's aim is to encourage the child freely to recall memories and perceptions of adverse experiences. Furthermore, the aim is to do this without introducing or suggesting any version of events that emanates from the practitioner (leading questions). Many children will be aware of the reason for the interview, either because they have previously expressed their concern or because the broad purpose of the interview has been discussed during a preparation phase. A single open-ended prompt from the practitioner is often sufficient to enable the child to start talking freely about areas of concern. This particularly applies to those children who have disclosed information previously (Sternberg *et al*, 1997). Some sample open-ended prompts are set out in Box 11.8.

Clearly, if children pre-empt the practitioner and launch into an account of their concern, it would not be appropriate to stop them or discourage them while they are spontaneously recounting memories. If

**Box 11.8** Prompts and questions to direct a child's attention to issues of concern

- Do you know why you are here today?
- I want to talk now about why you are here today.
- Tell me the reason you came here today.

this happens before there has been a chance to set out the ground rules for the session, these can be returned to at a later stage in the interview, if necessary (Poole & Lamb, 1998).

Sometimes these straightforward approaches do not lead to the child communicating anything. In these circumstances the practitioner may feel there is sufficient concern to justify further exploration, and some means will need to be found to explore these gently, without introducing any new information. We explore such situations next.

## Enquiry into suspected adverse experiences

There are circumstances when practitioners decide there is sufficient concern to talk to the child about possible adverse experiences. Examples of this include: where it has been decided, after a strategy meeting, that the child's situation does not fulfil criteria for a joint investigation (Department of Health *et al*, 1999, paras 5.31, 5.32); where there has already been an *Achieving Best Evidence* interview and a decision not to press criminal charges has been made, yet there is sufficient concern to justify further exploration. These are the grey areas, which appear to be quite common in practice. The approach that the practitioner follows depends on what kind of concerns led up to the current assessment. The following possibilities are quite frequently encountered:

- The child may have already spoken to someone about particular concerns.
- The child may be considered to be at risk of some form of adversity or maltreatment.
- The child may have been found to have a physical condition that raises the possibility of maltreatment (for example, unexplained bruising, sexually transmitted disease or anal bleeding).
- Behavioural change in the child may have led to concerns expressed by parents, teachers or some other adult.

Under separate headings below are some suggested phrases for managing the transition to an enquiry about adverse experiences. They are organised according to the mode of presentation and the origin of concern. Within each category, the questions progress from relatively open enquiries to direct questions.

## When the child has already disclosed information of concern

'I understand something may have happened that upset you [or scared you, or made you sad]. Please tell me every detail about what happened, from the beginning to the very end.'

'I understand that some things have been happening in your family [or school, another house, etc.]. Tell me about them.'

'I have spoken with your mum [or your teacher, etc.] and it sounds as though a lot of things have been happening in your family [or school, etc.]. Tell me about that.'

'Your mum said she had talked with you about some things that had upset you. Tell me about that.'

## Adult suspicion about a place or person

'Tell me about … [the place, person or time of incident causing concern].'

'Tell me who looks after you when your mum goes out. [Pause.] What things do you like to do with [name of baby-sitter, childminder etc.] … Is there anything that you don't like when [your baby-sitter] looks after you?'

'I've been talking to your mum and she told me she was worried about you [at a particular place or time]. Tell me everything about what happened.'

'Your mum told me that you get upset when Uncle John comes to stay at your house. Tell me about that.'

## At risk of harm

First, introduce general enquiry about the situation in which the child is considered to be at risk. This general enquiry would relate to school where the concern relates to bullying, or to punishment for wrongdoing where the concern is physical abuse in the home, or to family relationships or household arrangements, or likes and dislikes, where the concern is about possible sexual maltreatment within the household.

In other circumstances a child may have described some adverse circumstances and the practitioner is concerned about other possible forms of adversity:

'You've told me that [give summary of adverse events already disclosed, such as witnessing inter-parental violence, being bullied, experiencing physical or sexual abuse]. Have you been hurt [or upset or harmed] in any other way?'

'Has anybody done anything else to you that you didn't think was right'?

'Did anything else happen to you at ... [place or time of already disclosed incident]?'

'Did any other person hurt you?'

'Your [brother, say, or the name of different child about whom there is concern] has told me about some things that were happening to him. Tell me what you know about that ... [Then, after a pause] and he was worried about you?'

'Did anyone do something to you that you didn't think was right?'

'Did anything happen to you at ... [place or time of the abuse disclosed by another child]?'

## Inter-parental violence

Enquire about home, in general. Then use questions such as the following:

'What's the best thing about being at home?' followed by: 'What's the worst thing about being at home?'

'Your mum told me that she and your dad have been arguing – getting upset. Tell me everything about that.'

'Have you worried they might hurt each other?'

Or, for a younger child:

'Have you been worried that your mum might hurt your dad?' Then repeat with '... that your dad might hurt your mum?'

'Your mum told me that she had to go to the hospital [or doctor] after she had an argument with your dad. Tell me everything about that time.'

## Physical disease or change

'I've been talking to Doctor X. She told me that [brief reference to condition, using the child's own words, for example, you've had trouble going for a wee-wee, or a sore bottom, or pain when you go to the toilet].'

In the case of a young child with suspicious repeated urinary tract infections or a sexually transmitted disease:

'I've been talking to Doctor X. She told me that you've had to have some medicine [or tablets or injections] because of a problem in your bottom – can you tell me everything about that?'

## Behaviour change

*Enquiry directly about the child's symptoms (anxiety, depression, nightmares):*

'I hear you've been worrying a lot. Tell me all about that.'

'I hear you've had a lot of very scary dreams. Tell me what happens when you have them.'

'You've told me you're very depressed [or worried or upset] – tell me all about that.'

### Enquiry when child displays sexualised behaviour problems:

'Can you think about the time when you were playing like that with Fred? Tell me everything about that.'

Followed by:

'Have there been any other times when things like that have happened?'

Or:

'Has anybody done things like that with you'?

### Enquiry specifically concerning aggressive behaviour:

'I want to talk with you now about ... [an aggressive episode]. Tell me everything about that time.'

Followed by:

'Have there been other times when things like that have happened?'

'Do you know why that [aggressive episode] happened?'

'Have there been any things that have been upsetting you?'

'Has anybody done things like that to you?'

### Specific questions following deliberate self-harm:

'Do you know why that happened?'

'Have any things been upsetting you?'

Follow this with a general enquiry about school, friends, family members. For example:

'Sometimes young people hurt themselves [or take tablets] if they have something very upsetting that they have seen, or has happened to them, and they don't know how to talk about it. ... [Pause.] Has anything like that happened to you?'

Then, direct questions about the possibility of maltreatment may be used (see p. 138).

## Further approaches

If the above approaches do not result in a child providing an account that answers the question of whether or not he/she has experienced or witnessed adverse events, it may be appropriate to probe further. The aim is still to encourage the child to produce a free account and so it will be important to link any more directive probes with an open-ended invitation to the child to say more. Thus if the child says yes to any invitations, but especially the more directive ones, the next question needs to be along the lines of 'Tell me a bit more about that', or 'I think I understand, but just help me by telling me a bit more about that'.

One way of directing children further is to remind them of the interviewer's role. For example, the interviewer can preface an enquiry with the following phrase:

'My job is to talk with children about things that might have happened to them [might have seen; might have upset or harmed them].'

The interviewer can then continue by framing one of the questions selected from the above list, depending on the mode of presentation.

When the practitioner does this, it is important to avoid direct references to maltreatment, protecting children or to ensuring they are safe, unless of course the child asks the interviewer this. Equally, it would be suggestive to discuss issues of personal safety or comment on the conduct of adults. It can be helpful, however, to link the phrases suggested above with a reference to the importance of the child talking with the practitioner if something has happened.

Another line of enquiry that might be useful is as follows:

'Did anyone do something [to you or with you] that you didn't think was right?'

Before moving to more direct questions, particularly those that include reference to physical harm or sexual touch, it may be useful to return to more neutral matters and then approach the question of possible adversity again. An example of how this might be done is through discussing who is who within the family and where different people live. This can be a useful approach if concern has arisen about the behaviour of a household member. In younger children this can be done through drawing either a family tree or different homes in order to encourage such discussion (see Chapter 12). At some point, it will be possible to enquire about likes and dislikes, or to whom the child feels close and not so close. Any subsequent leads can be followed by with open-ended invitations to 'tell me more about that'.

Sometimes a child seems reluctant to communicate yet professional concerns remain. The choice is then whether to carry on or to arrange a further interview. This could be decided through having a short break, at the end of which the interview can either be recommenced or re-arranged for another time. It may be decided that greater preparation is required before proceeding. Alternatively it may be decided that it is best not to continue, while retaining the option for another assessment if there are further developments.

Plans will need to be made about managing the interim period. In particular, those to whom the child is likely to speak will require explicit instructions, advice and support during this interim time (for detail see Chapter 13). The aim of this action is to avoid contamination on the one hand, while providing the child with sufficient support so that an accurate and complete account of any concerns can be obtained at some stage in the future.

The emphasis on conducting only one interview, while under-standable in terms of preventing contamination of a child's account, has led to unhelpful urgency on the part of interviewers who think a one-hour single session is their only opportunity to obtain an accurate account from a child. This pressure is wholly unrealistic for young children, those with learning disabilities, those with communication impairments and those with psychiatric problems. Other children, too, may feel under such pressure that, although they are apparently prepared to communicate, they are simply unable to during the first session. Provided issues of preparation and the surrounding adult anxieties are contained, there is no reason to suppose that repeated interviews, per se, lead to inaccurate accounts (Powell & Thomson, 1997). If, of course, the repeated interviews are conducted inapprop-riately, for example if a predetermined 'answer' is relentlessly sought, the situation is very different (Ceci & Bruck, 1995). A repeat interview, therefore, if properly conducted, with due attention to what happens between sessions, is likely to be better than the practitioner becoming excessively anxious to 'extract' an account from a child in one single session.

## Direct questions

A final approach to exploring whether or not a child has suffered adversity is with more direct, focused questions and enquiries. With older children this will be in the form of questions, while with younger ones it may well occur in conjunction with indirect and non-verbal approaches to assessment, which are very useful aids for a variety of purposes within the interview and can be intermingled with periods of more direct talking (the use of indirect methods is considered further in Chapter 12). Those with communication impairments may be helped by the use of appropriate symbols, but broadly using the same sequence and gradation of enquiry from the most open-ended initially, through to more focused, direct questions, as follows:

### About place and time

'Has anything happened to you at ... [place or time of alleged incident]?'

'Did anything happen to you at ... [place, or actual time of abuse disclosed by another child]?'

### About physical assault

'Has anyone hurt you or hit you?... [Pause.] Either another young person, or an adult?'

### About domestic violence

'Have there been any times when your mum hit your dad, or dad hit mum?'

'Have you ever heard your mum and dad fighting?'

'Have you seen your mum hurt your dad?'

Repeat '... or your dad hurt your mum?'

### About bullying:

'Have you been hit or hurt by another child, either at school or on the way to and from school?'

'Have you been hurt in a sexual way by another child?' (For an older child.)

### About possible sexual assault

'Has anyone touched you on your body in ways that you didn't like?'

'Your mum said that you had some worries about being touched on private parts of your body. Tell me about that.'

'Has anyone touched the private parts of your body, and made you feel uncomfortable?'

'Did anyone, even a grown-up who you are close to, ever touch the private parts of your body?'

'I talk to a lot of children, and sometimes to children who have been touched on private parts of their body. It can help to talk about things like that. Has anything like that every happened to you?'

'Some children are touched on private parts of their body, sometimes by people they know very well. It can help to talk about things like that. Has anything like that ever happened to you?'

The last two examples involve permission-giving statements, initially, but end with a direct question. Questions of this kind are clearly potentially suggestive and would be of value therefore only if suspicion of adversity was high, and the nature of the concern being assessed was severe. Information yielded from such a direct question of this nature would have to be treated with caution. If a child answered such a question in the affirmative, the interviewer's response should be to revert to open-ended, neutral prompts. The key issue in terms of future validation of the child's communications would be whether the child merely reiterated the suggestion inherent in the question, or was enabled to respond in more detail to subsequent open-ended prompts.

Jones, D. P. H. (2003) *Communicating with Vulnerable Children*. London: Gaskell.

Sparing use of the occasional question of this nature is unlikely to lead to an error. This becomes a serious issue, however, if the entire tone of an interview is pressurised or hectoring.

## Further exploration

In many instances the child's predicament will have been clarified by the end of the second phase of the interview. It will either be clear that the child has experienced or witnessed adverse events, or professional concerns will have been allayed. In a proportion of cases, uncertainty continues, despite the professional's efforts. First, these latter situations are considered, then situations where concerns have been allayed and last those situations where concerns appear to have been confirmed.

### Continuing uncertainty

Sometimes interviews end in uncertainty or absence of clarity about the original concern that led to the assessment. These situations can be professionally frustrating, but it is preferable to close the session without having pressurised the child, than to be drawn through anxiety into a hectoring or coercive stance. Plans can be made for reassessment, review or for a further assessment interview with the child. A review of any impediments to successful communication may reveal useful pointers. For example, subtle issues of gender, ethnic or class differences between practitioner and child may have revealed themselves during the first in-depth interview, and these could inform a different approach to any subsequent assessment. Notwithstanding these considerations, children and parents, as well as other professionals, may well need advice as to what to do when faced with continuing uncertainty. It is essential to avoid imparting a sense of failure, or unwelcome expectations and pressure upon the child. The aim is to provide information and appropriate support. Box 11.9 lists some suggestions for practitioners when communicating with children in these uncertain circumstances. Parents, carers and other professionals may be helped by parallel advice. This is discussed in Chapter 13.

### Professional concerns allayed

In these instances, the interview with the child will need closure (see below) before the child returns home, in just the same way as interviews that reveal concerns (see below). The parent or carer will also need to be seen and the outcome and provisional impression fed back so that everyone is fully informed. Arrangements for follow-up or review, if necessary, will also need to be set out at this time. It may be that there will be other components of the core assessment of the child and family

---

**Box 11.9** Communicating with children when interviews end in uncertainty

If the interview ends in uncertainty as to whether the child has been victimised or not, the following are useful for the child and parent:

- Recognise the child's difficulty or distress, if present.
- Ask whether the child has anything further to say.
- Discuss with the child how to get help if it is wanted in the future (from social worker, docto:, counsellor, etc.).
- Separately discuss with the child how he/she can return to see the interviewer.
- Also discuss whether the child wants to see another person – and whether another person would be more helpful.
- There should be closure to the interview in the normal way.

---

situation to be completed, aside from the individual in-depth interview, and plans can be made for this at this point.

## Concerns about adversity confirmed

There will be a group of children who have revealed concerning experiences or events that they have witnessed. They will have responded affirmatively to some of the approaches outlined above. The decision for the practitioner at this point would be to decide whether it is most appropriate to continue the interview, in order to clarify the details of these experiences, or whether to make separate arrangements for the child to have an investigative interview in order to gather evidence for criminal proceedings (Department of Health *et al*, 1999; Home Office *et al*, 2002). This can be a difficult decision for the practitioner because it has to be made in the middle of an interview, and without the opportunity to confer with colleagues from other disciplines or supervisors. Furthermore, the child's revelations may not have been anticipated. The decision as to whether to proceed or bring the interview to a close and make arrangements for further work would include the following considerations:

- The practitioner's assessment of the session –
  - Is this a natural break point or not?
  - Is the child tired?
  - How long has the session lasted?
- What is the child's emotional condition – distressed, anxious? Or is the child relieved to be communicating with someone who is listening?
- The nature of concerns revealed thus far. Do the concerns constitute a very obvious potential crime (e.g. witnessing assault)

or clear-cut experience of maltreatment? In these instances the threshold for arranging an investigative interview would clearly be met and the current interview terminated as soon as reasonable from the child's perspective.

- An awareness of the local Area Child Protection Committee (ACPC) procedures for working together between agencies. Local procedures have often been agreed between agencies that set out trigger points and criteria for the holding of strategy discussions that may lead to the initiation of investigative interviews.

It may be possible to find an opportunity for a break, in which the practitioner can contact other colleagues on the basis of the above considerations. Clearly, it would not be appropriate to require a child to stop communicating when freely recalling adverse events. If it is decided to close off the in-depth interview and plan an investigative interview, then arrangements will need to be made for subsequent sessions with the child and immediate carers. There will remain children where further clarification about possible harm is indicated, once the practitioner has considered the above.

## Clarifying details about adverse experiences

If a child relays an account of abuse or a traumatic incident, it is likely that further details will be required. This can be about the events themselves or, in cases where there have been multiple incidents, clarification will be required about as many as it is possible to recall of these.

There is a wide range of details that may need to be asked about, depending on the individual case. In general, if detail is not spontaneously forthcoming, the following type of enquiry style is recommended:

'You told me about ... [summary using child's words ]. Tell me everything you can remember about that.'

'And then what happened?'

'Did anything else happen?'

'Has anything else happened?'

It may be necessary to find out whether anyone else has harmed the child if he/she has indicated one kind of harm:

'Did anyone else touch you [or hurt you, do things to you that you didn't like]?'

It may also be necessary to find out the frequency of the events described:

'Did that happen one time or more than one time?'

The question of multiple incidents frequently arises in physical and sexual abuse, and domestic violence. The interviewer will can be led by the child in many cases. In others it will be necessary to help the child to distinguish particular incidents. When establishing the detail of any events described by the child, the aim is to draw upon an event memory rather than a script memory, as the former are more reliable than the latter (see Chapter 2). Hence, any approach that directs the child's attention towards a particular event can be useful. Some commentators suggest focusing on the last incident first and then the first (if that can be recalled at all), perhaps followed by an incident that stands out because it happened at a particular place or at a particular time in the child's life, for example a birthday or holiday period. The interviewer should obtain an account of as many separate incidents as the child is able to recall. However, when children have suffered adversity many times each week over several years it is plainly not going to be possible to obtain an individual narrative about each incident. In such circumstances the questioning can be focused on one or two sample incidents that happened at particular places or that stand out in the memory of a child, perhaps because they were especially traumatic or involved some new form of abuse or experience of harm.

It is sometimes necessary to clarify the identity of people described by the child. This applies particularly to younger children, disabled children and those with an impairment, or where the child's circumstances are complex – with many individuals providing care for them or contact of other kinds. Some children have more than one person whom they call 'daddy', for example. It can be helpful to ask the child whether 'daddy' has another name, or what name mummy calls him, in order to clarify exactly whom the child means.

Professionals will need to gauge how safe the child is in the short and medium term. If the child has described maltreatment, it is necessary to determine whether the child is at risk of harm from anyone else besides the alleged abuser. In order to do this, further information will be necessary from the child as well as other family members. Has the child talked with anyone else about these adverse events, or attempted to do so? What was the response from the child's perspective? Has the child been threatened in any way, perhaps not to describe his/her experiences or what has been witnessed? Does the child feel safe with other people, family members or other potential carers? Did anyone else harm or threaten the child? Are there other siblings and in what way may they be involved? Who, if anyone, has helped the child in the past, and who does the child think might be able to help now? All this will need to be evaluated in conjunction with parallel assessments of the family.

Jones, D. P. H. (2003) *Communicating with Vulnerable Children*. London: Gaskell.

## Closing the interview

The closing phase of an assessment interview is all too frequently both perfunctory and too brief. However, this is a very important part of the session and one which can help orientate the child to the next steps, particularly if serious events have been described. The child is likely to need some degree of vindication, through recognition by the interviewer of the seriousness and difficulty of the issues that have been talked about. If the session has involved substantial expression of emotion, this should be openly acknowledged by the interviewer. It is perfectly reasonable for the interviewer to convey an appreciation and concern for the child's situation and difficult plight.

It is important to avoid congratulation, however, or phrases such as 'You have been very good'. Moreover, this is not the place or time for interviewers to express their personal point of view about the legality or morality of events described. Equally, interviewers must not promise that which they cannot deliver, or which may not be feasible. Thus discussion as to what might happen to an alleged abuser is not appropriate.

The child can be prepared for the immediate future, however. Next steps in treatment, further interviews or even placement, if known, should be discussed. It is important to be as honest and open with the child as possible. For example, children may ask whether they are going to see the interviewer again and the interviewer should be straightforward on this issue. It can be useful to check whether there are any residual concerns, using questions such as 'Is there anything else you think I should know?' or 'Is there anything else I should have asked you about?' In addition, it is important that children are asked whether they have any questions for the interviewer or anything else they want to say.

It is useful to discuss how the child can get help or assistance in the future, should it be required, particularly with an older child or teenager. Some young people are greatly assisted by being given a contact number for future reference. Confidentiality concerns often re-emerge at this point. Older children often ask what will happen to any video- or audio-tapes, records, notes and reports.

This phase of the interview is a key time for assessing the child's emotional status. Although some children are relieved to have communicated their experiences, others are markedly distressed after recalling and revealing adversity. Arrangements for helping the child will need to be considered, including what information parents, carers or the child's school need to have. There may be a requirement for therapeutic work, or further assessment of the need for this. Overall, the question of whether or not the child has experienced adversity needs to be set within a broader context of the child's overall needs and welfare status. It will be important for the practitioner to ensure that the scope of continuing enquiry and assessment is kept sufficiently broad to meet the child's needs.

Jones, D. P. H. (2003) *Communicating with Vulnerable Children*. London: Gaskell.

# CHAPTER 12

# Indirect and non-verbal approaches

## Observation

Observation is very important. Behaviour can be considered as a form of communication in itself, and may be intentional or not. Professionals who work with children have long valued the non-verbal aspects of children's communications. In part this is because young children are less able to communicate verbally than are school-age children and adolescents. Some non-verbal communication appears very direct in nature, such as the aggressive outbursts from a child who has suffered physical abuse or the sexualised behaviour demonstrated by some sexually abused children. The aggression of the neglected child is perhaps less direct, although no less serious or real in nature. Observed behaviour can be at significant variance, as well as congruent, with that which is expressed verbally. For example, one child's expressed wishes to return home contrasted dramatically with her parallel physical activity, which appeared to express extreme agitation (Jones *et al*, 1994).

Observed behaviours can, of course, be left to speak for themselves. Problems arise sometimes when behaviour is interpreted or meaning is ascribed to the observations made. Differences in value ascribed to the same behaviour can represent differing theoretical stances towards children's behaviour and development, but also represent the common values and purposes of different professional groups. For example, the meaning ascribed by different groups of professionals to children's play with anatomically detailed dolls has been examined (Everson & Boat, 1994). Social workers and psychoanalytically orientated therapists and psychiatrists were noted to be more likely to consider that the placing of two dolls together was likely to mean that the child had experienced or witnessed sexual activity than were a group of police officers, who were much more sceptical. Different professional groups place differing weight on verbal and non-verbal communications. For example, play therapists naturally emphasise non-verbal communication with children, whereas lawyers traditionally ascribe greater weight to verbal expression.

In the field of assessment, it is clear that care will be needed in making assumptions based on individual schemas of interpretation. We have already noted that the interviewer's assumptions play a significant part in the development of erroneous accounts of maltreatment. On the other hand, where therapeutic exploration of feelings is the primary function of the session with the child, there can be greater latitude with the use of interpretation and imputed meaning. For our purposes, however, we need to be explicit about the frame of reference used when reporting observations. Additionally, it is essential to separate observations themselves from the process of interpretation or ascribing

---

**Box 12.1** A schema for describing observations of behaviour

*Separation responses*
- How did the child separate from the parent?
- Was the child indiscriminate, or conversely unusually fearful?

*Physical appearance*
- Clothing, bruising, injury or impairment.

*Motor behaviour*
- Level of activity – restlessness, fidgeting, distractibility.
- Unusually slow or under-active?
- Changes in level of motor activity in relation to topics discussed.
- Unusual movements.

*Speech form and style*
- Clarity of speech.
- Changes in the speed or type of speech with changes in the topics being discussed.
- Unusual or idiosyncratic words.
- The use of words without apparent understanding of their meaning.
- Speech content.

*Social interaction*
- Interaction with the interviewer.
- Is the conversation appropriate or unusual?
- Is eye contact maintained?
- Is the child inhibited, aggressive, disinhibited or oppositional?
- What is the overall level of rapport and does the child maintain an appropriate distance and awareness?

*Affective (emotional) behaviour*
- Are there normal ranges of expected emotions?
- Are emotional responses appropriate to their content or focus of discussion?
- Are there any signs of emotions, such as sweating, rapid breathing, tearfulness, irritability, suspicion?
- Does the child seem fully aware and in touch with the surroundings and the context of the interview?
- Are there any unusual changes in mood, not explained by the interview's content?

*Level of consciousness*
- Child's alertness and awareness of surroundings.

---

meaning to them. This is especially important when assessments are likely to have an influence on major decisions for the child or family, for example in the context of family justice decision making.

Observations of non-verbal behaviour are important for the purposes of detecting emotion, assessing the level of attention and considering the congruence of non-verbal with verbal communications. Additionally, as noted above, any discrepancy between verbal and non-verbal communications can be an important source of information in itself. Much of the assessment of the child's developmental level is based on non-verbal communications and direct observations.

It can be helpful to organise the observations made. Box 12.1 offers an approach to this, based on recommendations by Angold (2000) and Yarrow (1960).

Once a child's observed behaviour has been described, using a schema such as that in Box 12.1, commentary or conclusions can be separately set out in any report that is written. This will permit a clear distinction to be made between observations and interpretations, which is likely to be important for later judgement and decision making.

Finally, it needs to be borne in mind that non-verbal communication is a two-way process. Interviewers communicate non-verbally as well as verbally. Much can be conveyed through one's facial expression, posture and gross actions, as well as subtle changes in inflection of voice. It is quite possible that children who have experienced traumatic events and threatening environments are more highly attuned to non-verbal communications of the adults with whom they come into contact than their more fortunate peers. Hence, practitioners in this area of work need to be careful about the expression of emotion and expectation (see Chapter 6).

# Toys and drawings

Play is a normal part of childhood in all cultures. It is seen particularly in the younger child, although in different forms is evident throughout childhood. Toys that represent people and objects from the child's world are a key ingredient of the young child's play activities. Play can be both playful and deeply serious. Representation, for example through drawing, has always formed a part of play. For those who work with children these observations are obvious, for they are an integral part of the activity of professionals from education, health and social agencies. They are also part of the parents' world, particularly before children enter school. The purpose of play has been studied extensively (Bornstein & Lamb, 1992). Its functions range from an activity that engenders confidence and familiarity with the objects within the child's world, through to providing the child with a medium for thinking about, making sense of and communicating thoughts, ideas and experiences. This latter aspect of play is particularly striking in children who are less verbal, through either developmental immaturity or disability.

Non-verbal activities are therefore traditionally a large part of the professional world of communication with young children. Toys and drawing materials have an immediate appeal to those faced with the very difficult task of communicating with young and less verbally able children. Does their use bring disadvantages, however? Is their use for assessment unsafe, because they encourage imagination and fantasy, so commonly associated with play activities? Does the encouragement of play inhibit the child's demonstration of verbal abilities within the interview?

Play materials might also lead children to provide inaccurate accounts because they link the toys and images with their general knowledge about how such objects can be used or how, in their experience, they are usually used (script knowledge), rather than encouraging a focus on specific events. Does play distract children from the main purpose of assessment interviews? Of even greater concern is the possibility that the materials themselves may be inherently suggestive of particular themes, such as abuse or trauma. Overall, then, do play materials lead to error, or increase the accuracy and completeness of accounts given by children with less-well-developed verbal abilities?

Before considering these issues further, we will consider the way in which play materials are used in this field. Toys and drawings can be used at a number of different points in interviews, and for different purposes.

- *To encourage rapport, and young children's comfort level and sense of ease within an interview*. This includes having toys available in a session and perhaps paper and markers. Dolls are also sometimes deployed for these purposes.
- *To direct the child's attention to an area of interest*. This includes presenting the child with materials such as dolls' houses, and small and large dolls, or other items that are in some way part of the interviewer's focus of concern. Technically, these are cues, where play materials are used as aids to memory retrieval. Cues include a full reinstatement to the original scene in which an alleged incident took place (environmental reinstatement), talking about items (verbal cues) or presenting selected representations of objects or the actual objects themselves, as toys or the genuine articles (object cues). Object cues are sometimes termed 'props'.
- *To label objects or parts of the body*. Here, the interviewer is using a drawing or a toy such as a doll to discover the child's words for particular items.

Jones, D. P. H. (2003) *Communicating with Vulnerable Children*. London: Gaskell.

> **Box 12.2** Issues involving the use of toys, drawings and props in interviews
>
> - Do they help or hinder?
> - If they do assist, are there any disadvantages in their use?
> - Is it possible to use 'Show me' instead of 'Tell me what happened?'
> - Are there distinctions between the use of drawings, toys and props?
> - What is the value of specific techniques such as the use of anatomical drawings or anatomically detailed dolls?
> - Can play materials be used safely?

- *To demonstrate.* Here, toys and materials are used to show the interviewer what happened when a verbal means of communicating proves difficult. This is sometimes used with doll figures, drawings or a more elaborate 'stage set', which might include furniture, rooms and figures.
- *To encourage enactment.* Here, the child is being permitted or encouraged to act out and demonstrate through play a particular theme (e.g. fearfulness, concern, alarm) or a sequence of events.

Play often encompasses a mixture of these aspects during an assessment. However, it can be useful to consider the way in which non-verbal techniques are being employed at any one time. What, then, are the issues facing practitioners when they use these familiar approaches with children during assessments? Box 12.2 summarises these.

# Research findings

## Overview of findings on toys and props

Findings from studies of the use of toys and props with children recalling a variety of events have proved helpful (Salmon, 2001; Pipe *et al*, 2002). They can be summarised as follows. Toys and a variety of physical props do assist children to recall information. Younger children, under the age of five years for example, are also more able to re-enact events using play materials. Hence, the increase in information provided about events is both verbal and, in younger children, non-verbally expressed. However, in many studies there is an increase in inaccurate information reported by children when toys are used. This has not happened in all studies and may be related to the way in which toys are used, rather than simply whether they are used or not. Furthermore, when interviewing children who may have experienced adversity, it is often unclear which toys and props to present to the child, because it may not be clear exactly what, if anything, has happened. Some of the studies have presented a wide variety of props to children in an attempt to explore these issues, whereas in practice most interviewers would use only a simple, single prop such as a doll figure (not anatomically detailed). The outcome of the studies on error has been mixed, however.

## Can children link toys to specific events?

A major issue, which receives surprisingly little attention, is whether children appreciate the link between the toy being offered and the incident being explored. More particularly, does the toy actually represent the real object in the way that the interviewer thinks it does? Nowhere has this been more explicit than in the field of anatomically detailed dolls. Interviewers imagined that young children thought that the dolls consistently represented specific named persons in the family, or indeed the child him- or herself. A series of very important studies examined these ideas (DeLoache, 1995). It was concluded that some young children, at least those of three years and older, are able to link a scale model to an actual room. However, the adult idea that children (say, under the age of four years) can use a doll as a representation of themselves or another person did not stand up well to experimental testing. This is not really surprising, because to have an object represent a person in real life involves a sophisticated degree of abstract imagining and thinking. It is unlikely that children as young as two and three would have this ability or, at least if they were developing it by this age, that they would have the ability to distinguish between when they were functioning in the abstract or were communicating real events. In essence, the interviewer is trying to communicate with young children, age four and younger, at just the time when the children themselves are having the greatest difficulty with understanding the use of symbols and how to make one object or thing represent another. It is small wonder then that children make errors when assessed at this time in their development, but equally no surprise that they should also be able, under some conditions, to communicate and express themselves using play materials.

## Children's drawings

Somewhat similar observations have come from studies of children's drawings. In general, five- and six-year-old children may be assisted by drawing when recalling events. They are able to talk more about the event when the interview includes drawing as well as an invitation to describe incidents that happened to them. However, drawing does not necessarily help young children, say aged three or four years.

Unfortunately, some interviewers are particularly inclined to use drawings and toy replicas as prompts with the younger children because these children say less about the events that have happened to them, and find it more difficult to describe events in detail, even if they can describe them in outline.

In many of the studies, the inaccuracies of young children were associated with other crucially important contextual factors, which are highly relevant for practitioners in the field. Inaccuracy occurred when, in addition to drawing, children were asked questions that were either misleading or suggestive.

## Indirect benefits

An important positive effect of drawing and the use of toy replicas is that they appear to make children feel more at ease and that the length of interviews is longer when they are used. These benefits have to be balanced with the potential deleterious effects on distraction and preoccupation noted by some commentators (Poole & Lamb, 1998, p. 183).

# Implications for practitioners

Overall, drawing and toy replicas can help younger children, under the age of six years, to communicate about events. They do this through parallel verbal means as well as through enactment. However, there can be problems. Inaccurate information may also be conveyed, and this is particularly problematic when the use of play materials is accompanied by suggestive styles of questioning. Additionally, interviewers should not assume that young children use toy replicas to represent items or events in the ways in which adults might imagine they do. This especially applies to two-, three- and four-year-old children, who are at the stage of developing their ability for symbolic representation at the abstract level required to perform a task like this.

It seems that extraneous toy replicas are especially problematic and can lead to errors in young children. This particularly applies to replicas that the interviewer thinks represent events that in reality did not form part of the child's experience. An example of this is where an interviewer introduces doll play with a bed and small figures in order to cue the child's memory, but on the false assumption that sexual abuse had occurred. Because beds and figures are a regular part of every child's life, children's play and speech while using these items might lead to erroneous conclusions by the interviewer.

The overriding conclusion from these studies is that toys and materials should, preferably, be thought of in the same way that we consider moving to directive questions among older children, once efforts to encourage free recall by open-ended prompts from a child have been exhausted. The use of toy replicas and drawing at this stage would, therefore, be a developmentally appropriate medium for communication at the point at which, in older children, focused or directive questions would be used. The exception to this may be their use with younger children, in an extended introductory phase of the interview, in order to build sufficient trust and rapport.

If toys and props are used, then it would seem prudent to keep them as limited in number as possible and to use them sparingly rather than having a large assortment available. As soon as sufficient rapport is established, it has been shown that verbal enquiry about the possibility of adversity is surprisingly well accepted even by four-year-olds (Lamb *et al*, 1998). This process can be facilitated by having a break after an introductory, rapport-gaining phase and then starting again, this time without toys and materials present while prompts are made in relation to issues pertaining to harm.

Adults frequently assume that children of four or five years will not be able to respond to verbal instructions or enquiry. Experience with a semi-scripted interview protocol has shown this to be incorrect for a significant proportion of children. Hence it may be that interviewers are generally too quick to reach for their familiar toys and play materials in their efforts to communicate with young or disabled children. Moreover, if, as is recommended in Chapter 11, the rapport phase of an in-depth interview becomes more important in its own right (and not merely restricted to the establishment of rapport, but also includes initial identification, communication of the ground rules, a time to practise communications and to illustrate how these ground rules work), then the unfocused use of toys and play materials is likely to diminish.

Are we able to draw distinctions between drawing, use of play replicas and the presentation of particular items such as anatomical drawings and anatomically detailed dolls? Drawings are used for different purposes, for example as a way of illustrating people doing things, to illustrate a particular theme, as free drawings, or to illustrate a particular point that has just emerged verbally. They are also used at different times during an interview, for example at the beginning, in order to encourage rapport between interviewer and child, in the early part of an in-depth interview, in order to focus attention on family members before asking direct questions, as an accompaniment to a direct enquiry about victimisation, or, finally, as a means of clarifying an event recalled by the child.

One of the advantages of using drawing is that direct eye gaze is temporarily averted, and at the same time the child's focus of attention is on drawing rather than on the interviewer's face. This may be a great help to some children, particularly when describing embarrassing or difficult information.

There are, however, concerns about using drawing as a rapport-gaining exercise (Poole & Lamb, 1998, p. 183), as noted above.

Nonetheless, drawing may be of value if the exercise of establishing rapport is wholly separated from enquiry about possible harm. Sometimes, with young children or disabled children, an extended evaluation of the child's abilities will be required, and because play and the use of drawing help interview sessions to progress without awkward pauses (Butler *et al*, 1995), the technique could be used, providing it is done with care. However, it would be probably wise, until further data are available, to avoid having pencil and crayon on the table as an introductory mode for every child, but rather to have them in reserve where rapport is especially difficult to establish.

Drawing may well assist children to describe further detail once they have disclosed, in outline, that some form of adversity has occurred. However, interviewers need to be careful to avoid suggestive questions at the same time as using drawing. In view of the uncertain effects of some combinations of drawing and questions, it would seem best to reserve the use of drawing for this purpose to that point in an interview where direct questions would normally be appropriate. In keeping with the advice for the use of directive questions (see Chapter 11), any disclosure of information through drawing should be paired with open-ended prompts to the child to say as much as possible about what has just been drawn.

Drawing can be very helpful in clarifying particular details of a child's otherwise fully verbal account. This can occur even in older children. For instance, the use of drawing to detail tablets or implements that are alleged to have been used in abusive acts has been very effective and, in individual cases, these details have been corroborated by crime scene investigations. The skill for interviewers remains to keep the individual child focused on describing a particular event, rather than that which usually happened (script memory) or that which might happen (hypothesis). In essence this is no different from spoken interviews, but commentators quite rightly caution that drawing and toys can be associated with the use of imagination and the expression of fantasy.

## Toy replicas

Broadly similar observations can be made about the use of object cues (life-size and toy replicas). Children are likely to be able to report more, but some of this information is likely to be added in error. The main benefit is seen in children of five and six years, whereas children of two and three years are less assisted by prompts in the form of toy replicas.

## Anatomically detailed dolls

The use of these dolls has been very thoroughly investigated from several perspectives and there are a number of helpful reviews of the research and their use in the field (Boat & Everson, 1988; Everson & Boat, 1994; Ceci & Bruck, 1995; Poole & Lamb, 1998). They have been extensively used in the USA, where much of the research has originated. They have been less used in routine investigations of possible sexual abuse in the UK. They cannot be recommended for routine use in assessment interviews for several, interrelated reasons. In the first place, they are probably theoretically flawed with respect to younger children due to the 'figurality of the symbolic representation' (DeLoache, 1995) in this age group. There is no convincing evidence that they help children more than verbal and other approaches that do not use detailed dolls (Lamb et al, 1996). This is a very important finding, because if there were evidence of benefit, even at the expense of some accuracy, a case could be made for their limited use in certain circumstances.

Another important finding is that anatomically detailed dolls increase error and particularly errors of commission, especially in younger children (i.e. children indicating or saying they have been touched when in fact they have not). It has also been found that the use of anatomically detailed dolls reduces verbal clarification and other forms of communication that are more likely to be accurate. It appears that the use of anatomically detailed dolls is especially problematic when combined with questions that are directive or suggestive. There is no evidence that the free play of sexually abused children with anatomically detailed dolls differs in a consistent and predictable way from that of non-abused children.

What about their use to name body parts? The obvious objection is that the overt nature of the dolls and their dissimilarity from dolls with which children normally have contact focus the child's attention on sexual matters. There is some evidence that this effect occurs, as reported by the mothers of three- and four-year-old children after a single interview with anatomically detailed dolls (Boat et al, 1990).

Is there, then, any place for anatomically detailed dolls? The only possible use that remains is for the clarification of acts of victimisation after a verbal account has been given, in children who are older than approximately six years of age and who do not have learning disabilities. From surveys, in the USA at any rate, this is the least likely use for anatomically detailed dolls. On present evidence, even if anatomically detailed dolls led to a disclosure of abuse, which was then followed by verbal questioning to clarify the account, one could not be sure about its veracity. It would seem safe, therefore, to restrict the use of anatomically detailed dolls to older children, and to use them only at the end of an interview, if at all, after other means of verbal and non-verbal communication have been tried.

## Anatomical drawings

Ready drawn anatomically detailed drawings (line drawings of male and female bodies), both front and back views, adult and child, are sometimes used to help children to communicate their words for body parts, to help them overcome their embarrassment or reluctance to use their own words for sexual body parts, and as an accompaniment to verbal disclosure. The research evidence is encouraging that the use of such drawings helps children to communicate. Sometimes this technique has been integrated into computer packages and forms the heart of a computer-aided interview scheme (Calam *et al*, 2000).

Similar observations to those made about drawing and toy replicas, above, apply to line drawings. That is, because a significant minority of children make errors when such techniques are used, great care must be taken with the type of accompanying questions. Hence the combination of line drawings with suggestive questions has been found to be problematic. Pointing to the diagram in the genital area while also asking children whether they have been touched in this part of their body can result in false reports. Although a majority of children will answer this question accurately, correcting the interviewer if wrong, or revealing that they have been touched if indeed they have, the problem for practitioners is that there is a minority who will make an error and say that they have been touched in a particular area when in fact they have not. This effect can be reduced, however, by careful pre-interview preparation. This is an important issue and emphasises once again the value of the introductory phase of interviews. It also underlines the importance for interviewers in all circumstances of adopting a neutral yet empathic stance towards the child.

There seems to be no harm in using line drawings to help children to identify body parts and to encourage them to give a fuller verbal account after they have made an initial disclosure suggesting that some form of maltreatment or adversity has occurred. If line drawings are to be used before any verbal or direct communication of harm from the child (possibly in situations where suspicion is high yet the child has appeared reluctant or finds communication difficult), then anatomically *neutral* drawings may be more appropriate. That is, the interviewer can have two sets of anatomical line drawings available for use: one set neutral and the other incorporating genitalia and breasts.

## Summary

Box 12.3 summarises the principal practice points from this chapter.

**Box 12.3** Summary practice points for the use of toys, drawing and props

- Observation is a key component of any assessment session with a child. Non-verbal communication can confirm verbal communication or may suggest new avenues for assessment. The description of observations should be kept separate from commentary upon it.
- Drawings and toy replicas have a place in interviewing and can assist children to communicate events that they have experienced.
- There are risks of error attached, which can be lessened by preparation, and by the interviewer taking care to avoid any accompanying suggestion when using toys and drawing.
- Anatomically detailed dolls do not help children to communicate and may lead to significant error. Their usefulness is very restricted.
- Ready drawn anatomical line drawings can be of assistance, especially after an initial disclosure from the child that harm has occurred, provided they are used with care. Neutral line drawings are more appropriate for initial enquiry.
- Disclosure of new information through the use of drawings and cues should be linked to open-ended invitations for further detail to be recalled spontaneously.

Jones, D. P. H. (2003) *Communicating with Vulnerable Children*. London: Gaskell.

# CHAPTER 13

# Advice for parents and carers

## First concerns

Parents are usually the first people to whom children turn if they have been victimised. Children may not do so if they are uncertain of their parent's support, or if they detect divided loyalty, or of course if any parent figures are involved in the abuse or maltreatment of the child. We know surprisingly little about these first communications that children have, but their quality is likely to have a significant influence on the accuracy of children's subsequent communications. It is known that parents report feeling shocked and rendered less able to function than normal when faced with their child suddenly disclosing maltreatment. Strong emotions are evoked in parents (Sharland *et al*, 1996). Most parents will not have time to seek advice before responding to their child's disclosures. However, in other circumstances parents may harbour initial suspicions and ask for professional help with how to proceed. Naturally, if concerns are specific enough, the professional's task will be to encourage appropriate referral, if necessary offering to facilitate that process in partnership with the parent. However, professionals are often faced with parents who have concerns that their child may have been maltreated, or otherwise traumatised, yet with insufficient basis to recommend referral. Would any specific advice be helpful? If so, what might this consist of? The suggestions offered below are based on the idea that the parent has a delicate balancing job of, on the one hand, supporting their child, while, on the other, also avoiding unhelpful influences that might distort the child's memory of events.

The first task of the professional is to explore the basis for the parent's suspicions. Sometimes, from a professional perspective, alternative explanations other than maltreatment are quite feasible to explain the parent's worries. However, the basis for concern is important to clarify, including the exact timing and sequence of events and concerns that the parent has noted. It can often be helpful to stress the importance of maintaining a line of communication between parent and child, especially if the child appears to be struggling to convey confusing feelings and adverse experiences. Helping the parent to appreciate the

**Box 13.1** Advice professionals can give to parents who are concerned their child may have been harmed or traumatised

*An open mind*
- Try to keep an open mind as to what may or may not have happened to your child, while allowing your child time and space to tell you anything they need to.

*Listen but don't question*
- Let your child tell you what they wish to, in their own words and their own time.
- Don't ask questions such as 'Did he touch you down there' or 'Did he hit you for doing that?' Leave that for the social worker or other professional to find out about.

*Support*
- Give your child as much emotional support as you can and let them know that you are there to listen. Say you will not be upset, or distressed or angry with them, whatever they wish to say to you.
- Do not put pressure on your child because they may find this too much, and if they do want to talk to you, they may be inhibited. Also, it will make it difficult to protect your child properly in the future, unless your child is able to speak in their own words.

*Stay calm*
- Try and keep as calm as possible, even if you do not feel this way inside. Otherwise your child may notice your reaction and worry so much about you, that they bottle up their own feelings, and don't communicate their concerns.

*Keep a record*
- If your child does say anything that concerns you, write it down as soon as possible afterwards. Do everything possible to remember your child's words, and your own, and to describe the circumstances in which they talked with you.

*Obtain further help*
- You can get further advice and help from the following number: [insert local number(s) here]

child's possible struggle and difficulty can be a useful way of keeping communication open. The importance of avoiding pressurising the child should be stressed to the parent. This can be explained in terms of children's raised anxiety if they perceive the parent to be pressurised, anxious or demanding. It can also be framed in terms of the difficulties that professionals will have in the future when planning for the child's safety and welfare, if information has been drawn from the child under duress or pressure.

This is often a very delicate conversation to have with anxious parents when they, in turn, may be in need of support for their own distress and anxiety. Nonetheless, it can be very helpful to parents if the professional emphasises the importance of retaining an open mind as to what may lie behind the child's behaviour. Also, their anxiety may be partially allayed by the parents knowing that continuing support and review are available, in the light of any further information. If the child appears to be distressed, the parent's role in providing support is of crucial importance to the child's well-being, even though the parent may feel somewhat emotionally unavailable. It will, of course, be necessary to review the child's safety with the parent and to respond as necessary. It may be helpful to provide parents in this situation with written material to back up any advice given orally. Box 13.1 offers a framework for such advice.

## Advice during the process of assessment

There is likely to be a delay between an initial assessment and any subsequent in-depth interview, if a decision is made to proceed in this way. Sometimes this will be a matter of hours, but frequently several days pass while appropriate preparations and professional planning occur. Detailed plans about how best to communicate may be necessary, especially for children with particular needs or communication impairments.

Very little is known from field-based research studies as to what happens during this period in typical cases, or what influence the management of this interim period has on the future reliability of children's accounts. However, extrapolating from the concerns about children's suggestibility (Ceci & Bruck, 1995), it would certainly be wise to pay attention to this period, in order to prevent untoward negative effects on the child and their testimony. This particularly applies to younger children and children with learning difficulties, who may be especially prone to be influenced by the perceived expectations of the adults who are caring for them. Children are also likely to be affected, and their security perhaps undermined, by their observations of their carer's mental state. Thus, considerable demands are placed on adult carers in this situation (Sharland et al, 1996), which are frequently not fully appreciated by the professional community. They may well be in a state of shock and personal distress because of the recent revelation of the possibility of maltreatment, and at the same time are being required to support the same child through a key period. Not only that, but we ask them also to refrain from doing what most parents feel inclined to do in these circumstances – to ask questions and learn everything there is to know about any possible adversity experienced by their child.

Hastening in-depth interviews is unlikely to be the answer, because one of the strong messages from a child's perspective is concern about

---

**Box 13.2** Ingredients of parent preparation

• Emotional support.
• Practical advice and information.
• Discussion of parents' role in forthcoming interviews.
• Discussion about child's need for confidentiality.
• Continuing advice about the response to the child's concerns/allegations.
• Discussion concerning what their child has been advised.
• Resources for further advice/support.
• Advice to refrain from intrusive or over-eager enquiry with their child.
• Obtaining information about any special communication needs that the child may have.
• Requests for information about the names of key family members and other people to whom the child may refer during the forthcoming assessment.

---

the speed of the professional reaction and the fact that they are not involved with what is happening to them (Wade & Westcott, 1997). Parents feel similarly (Sharland *et al*, 1996). In contrast, it has been demonstrated that preparation helps produce more accurate and complete accounts (Saywitz *et al*, 1991). Hence, although immediate assessment seems an attractive solution, it is probably inadvisable if the overall objective is to obtain reliable accounts of children's experiences. For this reason, considerable effort needs to go into preparing the child and immediate carer, and any other adult involved, for the process. At the same time, it gives the interviewers more time to prepare, consider and plan for any special needs that the child may have.

Central messages to convey to parents and carers are to emphasise the crucial value of their support of the child, while emphasising the importance of their retaining an open mind as to the possibilities of maltreatment, and advising them of the dangers of zealous or intrusive enquiry with their child. In order to do this, parents need support and information as well as understanding of their own likely mental state and distress. Box 13.2 sets out the items to cover in such advice. Children similarly require preparation.

## When uncertainty persists

Some assessments end in continuing uncertainty. These situations can prove especially difficult for professionals to manage. However, both child and parent or carer (or indeed teacher if the concern arose in school) will need advice as to what to do. The aims are to prevent an atmosphere of undue pressure or expectation on the child, or to impart

      Jones, D. P. H. (2003) *Communicating with Vulnerable Children*. London: Gaskell.

---

**Box 13.3** Advice for parents, in uncertain circumstances

If an interview ends in uncertainty as to whether any harm has occurred or not, the following points are useful to convey:

- The child has tried to communicate, but some children simply cannot.
- The child may have been abused or harmed, but equally may not have been. We simply do not know.
- Let the child take his/her own time and not feel pressurised.
- Emphasise the importance of avoiding intrusive questions or pressure.
- However, keep a line of communication open – 'You can talk to mummy whenever you want: just say so and we'll find a good time'.
- Discuss the fact that the child may be unable to talk with the parents for fear of creating distress in them or because the child feels guilty. Advise parents against raising questions about this; it is better that they merely understand and be aware of it.
- Advise parents to record any conversations they have with the child immediately after they have happened (situation, and all questions and answers that can be recalled).
- Advise as to where to obtain further advice and support, including how to contact the interviewer again.
- Clarify arrangements for follow-up.

---

a sense of failure. By contrast, the aim is to provide a supportive environment in which, should the child wish to disclose any information, he/she is able to do so. Advice to the parent or any other adult could include the items listed in Box 13.3.

# CHAPTER 14

# Epilogue

It is tempting to repeat the messages in preceding chapters and summarise them for added emphasis in this chapter. Instead, three new areas are selected for final mention, because they are crucial to effective practice. These are a framework for analysing information, training, and future directions for practice development.

The emphasis in this book so far has been on effective practice that enables children to talk about adverse events. The proposition advanced is that evidence-based good practice both helps children to communicate and results in more accurate and complete accounts from them. Such accounts, it has been argued, enable better and more informed decisions to be made about children's lives and their families. This is the central tenet of this book. However, there are additional points that contribute to good practice in this area. The management of practitioner bias and presupposition extends beyond direct working and communicating with children, into analysis and decision making. It has already been stressed that continuing professional development is essential for good practice (Chapter 6). Hence, some observations about training are noted below. Finally, the chapter ends with future directions that are likely to show promise in the near future.

## A framework for analysis

A practitioner has to evaluate the outcome of a session after talking with the child, and place the information obtained alongside other relevant information, in order to make a decision as to whether the child seems to have suffered harm or is likely to do so in the future. The ultimate truth, or otherwise, of an account of harm to a child is a matter for a relevant court to make a finding on. However, quite separately from the legal process, social services, police and health professionals often need to make a decision about whether there is sufficiently convincing clinical evidence to decide whether a child has suffered harm. There is no single test of this and instead we have to analyse the information before us in order to make a decision about whether the case is sufficiently convincing, from our particular professional perspective. We then base action upon this. Subsequent steps can range from making a decision that the child has not suffered any form of harm, to a conclusion that the situation is uncertain and

Jones, D. P. H. (2003) *Communicating with Vulnerable Children*. London: Gaskell.

requires further assessment, or that the child's safety needs to be assured.

Just as it is crucial to keep presupposition and bias from the practice of talking with children, so too is it helpful to ensure that such tendencies are kept in check during the subsequent analysis of the information obtained from a child, because in this process, too, there is the potential for error. Having a framework through which to consider the information can help to counteract the tendency to place an inappropriate degree of emphasis on one particular aspect of what the child said.

There have been several descriptions of systematic approaches to 'validation' within the field of child sexual abuse. Sgroi *et al* (1982) emphasised the need for a sound knowledge of the dynamics of child sexual abuse, good interviewing skills and an ability to interpret behaviour and any physical signs that were obtained during the investigation. These authors divided the process of validation into assessment of the child's behaviour, the results of the interview with the child, assessment of credibility, any physical indicators of abuse and findings from medical examination. Faller (1984) also considered the question of validation and emphasised the importance of observing an emotional response that was consistent with the nature of any maltreatment described, the presence of any idiosyncratic memories surrounding any assault described, the importance of the child's viewpoint of the event and his or her statements to other children, play and abnormal knowledge of sexuality as helpful indicators. Jones & McGraw (1987) described their practice of analysis and decision making in their detailed examination of false allegations of sexual abuse. They stressed that absolute measures of truthfulness were not available and emphasised multidimensional approaches to analysis that placed accounts from children along a 'continuum of certainty'.

Also in the field of child sexual abuse, Heiman (1992) considered that a multidimensional decision-making process should include: a consideration of the history of any symptoms, the verbal account given by the child, the phenomenology of the child's experience of abuse, the child's presentational style and the presence or absence of any corroborating evidence. Jones (1992) suggested that the following areas were useful to consider when making decisions about possible sexual abuse cases: the child's account and behaviour during interview; his or her behavioural and emotional state both before and after assessment; the process of disclosure; any prior accounts or expressions of concern; family factors; and the presence of physical or physiological evidence. He suggested that primary importance should be given to the account of the child. He stressed that such a system should not be taken as a method of assessing truthfulness but merely as a framework through which to make clinical decisions. Such a framework was intended to permit a clinician to assess 'the degree of certainty' that could be applied to an individual case (Jones & McGraw, 1987; Jones & Seig, 1988; Kolvin *et al*, 1988).

Horowitz *et al* (1995) discussed the need to establish 'ground truth' in relation to child sexual abuse when considering criteria for the inclusion of subjects in research studies. Following a review of the literature, these authors proposed nine sources of information that could contribute to a decision about 'ground truth', together with procedures for assessing their validity. These sources of information were: medical evidence; confessions; witness statements; confessions about coaching; serial victim statements; recantations; polygraph examinations; physical or material evidence; and statement assessment.

The framework used by the National Children's Advocacy Centre (Carnes *et al*, 1999) comprises the following areas for analysis: disclosure factors; the presence of attempts made by the professional to decrease potential suggestion; specific details recounted by the child; an assessment of whether the account is consistent with the child's developmental status; any emotion expressed by the child while talking; results of behaviour checklists; presence of any corroborative information; consideration of motivational factors for the child's account; and any other alternative explanations for the child's account.

Poole & Lindsay (1998) have examined two traditional approaches to the assessment of the accuracy of young children's reports of child sexual abuse: the indicator approach, where the emphasis is on identifying characteristics that distinguish true from false reports; and the assessments approach, which compares reports of possible sexual abuse from children in different interview conditions. Their detailed review critically analyses the evidence in each of these two traditions for 'commonly cited aphorisms about how to discriminate between true and false reports'. Their helpful review should lead to a great deal of caution among practitioners when making conclusions about the truthfulness or otherwise of allegations. This is because the ability to distinguish sharply between true and false reports is substantially less than many commentators would assert. For specialists undertaking core assessments and in-depth interviews with children, their review is helpful when analysing or attempting to make sense of information obtained from a child.

The following framework for analysis is proposed, based on the approaches considered above.

## The child's account

The child's account can be assessed with regard to explicit detail of the alleged harm. Overall, younger children are not able to relate as much

Jones, D. P. H. (2003) *Communicating with Vulnerable Children*. London: Gaskell.

detail as older ones. However, the more detail that is recalled, the more likely it is that the account refers to the child's own experience, especially if it is considered unlikely that an individual child could have gained such detailed knowledge without personal experience of the event in question. However, care has to be taken to consider the unfolding of the child's account and the nature of the influences that might have borne upon it. Poole & Lindsay (1998), quoting Bruck et al, emphasise that in experimental studies, while the consistency of the accounts did differentiate true from false, this became less potent over time if children were repeatedly interviewed. This was because false stories took on additional qualities that made them seem more like true narratives.

Nonetheless, the words and sentence formation of the account should be congruent with the expected developmental status of the child. For example, one five-year-old child appeared to make a false recantation of her previously made allegations of child sexual abuse. When she was asked why the sexual abuse had stopped, some 18 months previously, she said 'because it was inappropriate'. This phrase appeared to indicate its adult rather than child origins. It has also been noticed, however, that some children's accounts can appear unbelievable because they adopt the language used by case-workers, therapists and others around them. Reference to the early statements of the child can help to establish a better basis for assessing the accuracy of the child's statement, which emphasises once again the importance of full records of all the accounts that children have made about any alleged incidents of harm.

It can also be useful to examine the child's account for signs of unique or distinguishing detail. This can be found both in accounts of any individual experiences of victimisation or in unrelated recollections. For example, some sexually abused children describe smells and taste associated with sex. Similarly, children who have witnessed severe assaults or the murder of a parent have described the distinctive smell of blood. One four-year-old boy described the feeling of rectal stretching while being anally penetrated as 'I felt like I wanna go pooh-pooh'. In addition, children sometimes describe in great detail matters which were not essential to the assault being described, such as the distinguishing features of a room, bed or clothes that the child was wearing at the time. One three-year-old girl said, 'I had my panties on backwards'.

A child's statement can also be searched for evidence of a child's perspective of any incident of assault, in contrast to that which might be expected to come from an adult or from a third party. Such a 'child's eye view' of an alleged incident would seem especially hard to account for through suggestion. However, once again this may be possible after repeated suggestive and especially coercive interviews.

Jones, D. P. H. (2003) *Communicating with Vulnerable Children*. London: Gaskell.

The emotion expressed by a child during an interview is usually congruent with the events being described, in genuine cases. It is quite feasible that a child will experience one part of an aversive or abusive situation as more offensive or emotionally striking than another. Furthermore, this differential may not coincide with the adult practitioner's assumption as to what was probably the most severe or worst experience for the child. Children may also display signs of acute anxiety at key points during an interview or avoid particular areas of inquiry. Sometimes, among children who have been sexually abused, sexualised behaviour is evident during the session itself. These and similar expressions of emotion tend to be associated with genuinely experienced accounts more than with false or erroneous ones. However, once again these distinctions may become less sharp over time, particularly in the presence of serial, suggestive interviewing by parents or professionals.

It is useful to consider whether the child's account is given in an apparently rehearsed or packaged manner, or with the emotion that might be expected. However, even here practitioners need to be aware of the great variation in the emotion that children express at different ages in relation to similar events.

How the child provides the account during an interview can be a useful source of information. For example, is the child's account forthcoming after the slightest cue from the interviewer or is there a degree of difficulty, reserve or hesitancy? Is the emotion expressed genuine or does it seem contrived or hollow in its manner of expression? Is the child bland, unemotional and seemingly little perturbed when revealing memories of adverse experiences? It can also be useful to see whether children recall how they felt at the time of the alleged incident. For example, did the child feel sad, frightened, angry or guilty?

The nature, type and pattern of any abusive events described by the child can also be of assistance in the assessment of accuracy. For example, in the field of sexual abuse, the clinical pattern frequently does not involve penetrative acts but may be restricted to oral or sexual touching. The context and timing can provide useful clues as to accuracy, too. Physical assault can occur at particular times in response to particular triggers, such as the child's misdemeanours or following arguments between parents. In cases of sexual abuse it is common for there to be several incidents over time, particularly in abuse by persons known to the child. Frequently there is progression of one sort of sexual act to another over a period of months or years.

In cases of sexual abuse an element of secrecy is frequently found. For example, the perpetrator may say 'This must be our special game – don't tell anyone, not even your mum'. Children are sometimes coerced into activity and threatened not to tell anybody. They may be told that harm will come to them or that they will be removed from the people

Jones, D. P. H. (2003) *Communicating with Vulnerable Children*. London: Gaskell.

they love if they do reveal the 'secret'. Of course, such coercion or threats are not always evident in initial interviews, particularly if a child is too fearful to talk freely.

There are sometimes other, much less common features of accounts of sexual or physical abuse that can assist decision making about accuracy. These can include descriptions by children of sadistic activity, or involvement with pornography. Sometimes these elements can be corroborated through timely police investigation.

## The child's behaviour and emotional state

The child's behaviour during the period of alleged maltreatment may show features in common with other children who have experienced similar events. There is no one set of symptoms that are reliably associated with a particular adverse experience. As has been stressed (Chapter 4), there is a great variety in children's emotional behaviour and responses to particular kinds of events and adversities. The search for a particular syndrome or distinguishing set of emotional and behavioural responses that will provide a reliable indicator of a child having experienced a particular event is likely to be fruitless. However, the presence of certain behaviours and emotional responses may be in keeping with the child's account of events, even if not indicative. For example, a child describing severe inter-parental conflict in the home may have been displaying significant behavioural problems, talking about these experiences. Similarly, some sexually abused children display sexual behaviour or developmentally inappropriate and unexpected sexual knowledge.

## The process of disclosure

There is considerable debate about the manner in which children disclose experiences of sexual abuse (Chapter 7). However, it can be useful to attempt to trace the manner in which a child's account has unfolded and what influences there were upon this process. While it is clear that there is great variation between children, an examination of the process may be useful when assessing accuracy. Key questions are 'Whom did the child tell?' and 'What motivated the child to do so?' Is the process of disclosure in this particular case understandable, given the pressures known to have been bearing down on this child not to tell? A child may have made a statement to other people before any in-depth interview. Children quite frequently talk to other children, or perhaps to neighbours, parents or teachers, before they are formally interviewed. The content of the accounts given to these people may be usefully compared with that obtained from an in-depth interview.

This raises the issue of consistency between different statements made by a single child. There is usually, in truthful accounts, consistency of the core elements of the child's account, but there may be some variation in more peripheral aspects. Thus, the question of consistency is not an all-or-nothing matter. It may vary with the degree of personal poignancy of the particular experience for that child. Similarly, violent elements of coercion or threatening behaviour by a perpetrator can be extremely frightening for the child, who may consequently suppress these elements for a longer period than other aspects of the harm being described. This can give rise to an air of apparent inconsistency in a child's account of harm. However, running through the account would be a consistent thread of harm described. In contrast, false statements are often made with monotonous consistency from the beginning and show little variation over time.

## Prior accounts or expression of concern

It is often helpful to review any previous accounts of possible harm that the child has made, perhaps of an incomplete or indeterminate nature. Also, concerns may have been expressed by relatives or neighbours, which can be all considered alongside the child's account, to look for potential congruence or an explicable pattern.

## Witness statements

It can be useful to assess any accounts and statements from other children or adults who are either involved or were in the household at the time, or who may otherwise have a view on the alleged incidents. Clearly, the motivation or level of involvement of the witness will affect the weight attached to the account (Horowitz *et al*, 1995). However, sometimes other children have actually seen harm occurring to the index child, or have some knowledge of the activity occurring within the family. Sometimes, also, the index child will have shared experiences of adversity with a brother or sister.

## Information from a family history or assessment

In cases where harm is alleged to have occurred within the family, the biographies of other family members and the history of the family can provide helpful and supportive information. The track record of the adults with regard to violence, inter-parental conflict, alcohol or substance misuse and criminality may be in keeping with the account of harm provided by the child in an in-depth interview. There may also be a pre-existing history of neglect or other forms of maltreatment, or of harm having occurred to other children within the family, all of which may be placed alongside the current account from the index child. The history of caretaking and child–parent attachment may provide further information that can assist the practitioner in an

Jones, D. P. H. (2003) *Communicating with Vulnerable Children*. London: Gaskell.

assessment of the accuracy of the child's account. It may also be possible to assess the degree of general dysfunction within the family; if so, this may provide further data to support or detract from the child's statement (Madonna *et al*, 1991).

## Medical evidence

Medical evidence of physical abuse can be extremely helpful in evaluating the accuracy of the child's account. Nonetheless, in the field of sexual assault, many children show no abnormal findings. Similarly, non-abused children reveal a range of findings that could be confused with abuse if they are not carefully evaluated. Additionally, the examination techniques themselves can influence the findings. The dimensions of the hymenal and anal orifices may give grounds only for suspicion, but signs such as tears in the genital area, pregnancy and the presence of sperm and blood enable a conclusion about sexual abuse to be made with more certainty.

## Physiological measures

Physiological correlates of truthfulness, such as the polygraph examination, are the subject of controversy, with strong advocates for both their value and lack of utility. At present a properly conducted polygraph report may be a useful adjunct but is unlikely to be determinative.

# Training

It is clear that training is essential but there is considerable difficulty in identifying what that training should comprise and how it should be delivered. If the perspective taken in this book is valid, then training needs to be conceptualised differently depending on the target group of professionals involved. That is, training approaches that might be relevant for those conducting in-depth interviews and undertaking comprehensive assessments of children are likely to be very different from those of practitioners who need training in how to communicate best with regard to first responses and in initial assessments (Chapters 9 and 10). There is no published work on training with regard to these latter circumstances, at least specifically that which relates to talking with children by, for example, teachers, health visitors or youth workers.

In the absence of any specific research it seems reasonable to attempt to ensure that the recommendations for practice outlined in Chapters 9 and 10 become incorporated into general child protection training programmes that are designed to induct front-line practitioners in non-specialist settings in social care, health and education. These child protection introductory training events often include information and discussion about how to respond to initial concerns presented by children, and so these would provide an excellent opportunity for very specific guidance about how to talk with children and respond to initial concerns without compromising any future assessment or investigation that may be required. Generally, practitioners express considerable anxiety about how to respond to initial disclosures of concern, especially when they are least expecting a child to talk to them. Practitioners often feel ill equipped and at the same time extremely anxious that they may compromise any future work that may be required with the child and family. It is proposed here that giving practitioners who work with children every day some straightforward guidelines about how to respond effectively and the things to say, as well as questions and approaches to avoid, would be of great value.

More information is available about training in relation to in-depth interviews with children. The consistent finding has been that improved knowledge does not necessarily result in better practice, particularly with respect to avoiding leading questions and adopting more open-ended methods when talking with children (Lamb *et al*, 1998; Aldridge & Cameron, 1999; Freeman & Morris, 1999; Jones, 1999; Orbach *et al*, 2000; Sternberg *et al*, 2001). This finding even applies where the training has been extremely well planned and educationally sophisticated in delivery (Aldridge & Cameron, 1999). In the field-based studies of Lamb and colleagues (Lamb *et al*, 1998; Orbach *et al*, 2000), when practitioners used scripted introductions to in-depth interviews with children they used fewer leading questions during that introductory section and more open-ended invitations to the children; however, these gains were lost as soon as the interviewers were free to return to their 'natural' style and were no longer required to use a protocol. This led Lamb and his colleagues to recommend a semi-structured interview protocol for the entire interview, in forensic interviews with children.

Other commentators have drawn attention to gaps in the philosophy and content of training programmes for in-depth interviews. For example, Hendry & Jones (1997) pointed out that training programmes that have crowded syllabuses often fail to cover disenfranchised, target groups of children, such as disabled children, as well as neglected yet essential aspects of practitioner behaviour, particularly with respect to what they term 'anti-oppressive' practice.

Davies *et al* (1998) used principles derived from health service audit, and drew upon the views and experiences of practitioners themselves to illuminate gaps in the provision of training for those interviewing children in forensic settings. This audit stressed that knowledge-based training on its own was insufficient to meet practitioners' needs. They recommended that initial, foundation training needed to be followed up

Jones, D. P. H. (2003) *Communicating with Vulnerable Children*. London: Gaskell.

with a second tier, which would seek to promote self-reflection, evaluation and performance enhancement of practitioners.

Taken together, these findings underline that a short intensive training course over one or two weeks is not the most effective way of training practitioners to interview children, particularly in forensic settings. It is quite clear from the results of the studies on effectiveness, as well as from surveys from practitioners themselves, that a more extended approach to long-term performance review and enhancement is required. One recommendation has been for follow-up advanced training courses (Davies *et al*, 1998; Aldridge & Cameron, 1999). It is probable, though, that these advanced or secondary courses will need the extra ingredient of continuing professional development and detailed review of actual interview practice if they are to meet practitioners' needs.

We have found locally that the best way of doing this is through small-group peer review, using video-taped segments of key areas of concern for practitioners, as well as hearing detailed accounts of exchanges during interviews and problems arising from these. The accent is on mutually supportive problem solving, as opposed to an overtly critical environment. Such a group should be able to provide ideas and be constructive and imaginative in assisting one another to address problems identified. However, in this author's experience, such activity is frequently seen as a luxury, to be put to one side when the pressures of case demands and intake take over. There would seem to be a need for a culture change at the organisational level so that such continuing professional development is regarded as essential to safe practice, rather than merely optional extras, 'if you have the time'.

While awaiting the outcome of more definitive studies, the ideal mix would seem to be an initial short course of training, to be followed up with some form of advanced training module, but combined with small-group peer audit and review of practice and adequate supervision. This is what appears to be required for practitioners conducting effective in-depth interviews with children. It is hard to see how this could be achieved without recognition of the specialisation involved in undertaking such interviews with a diverse group of children who present for assessment. However, to settle for less is to accept the current unsatisfactory state of affairs. The message from careful evaluations of training programmes is unequivocal: short introductory training programmes are insufficient to lead to the improvements of practice that are essential for evaluating the welfare status and protection of vulnerable children.

## Future directions for practice development

Practitioners in the field continually look for methods to improve their ability to assist children to communicate effectively during in-depth interviews. These difficulties are brought into relief by the problems involved in undertaking in-depth interviews with young children and those who have learning disabilities or particular communication or sensory impairments. Children and young people with severe mental health problems, but who also are attempting to communicate experiences of victimisation, also present major challenges for practitioners. The useful lessons for practitioners that have emerged from research on children's suggestibility (Ceci & Friedman, 2000) need to be extended to a more diverse group of children, such as those with significant disability or impairment. Similarly, practitioners would be helped by more information about the advantages and disadvantages of using different forms of indirect and non-verbal styles of communication among diverse groups of children. For example, just how suggestive or otherwise different forms of drawing and enactment are, and whether computer-aided approaches to in-depth interviewing are safe or not (Calam et al, 2000). Are semi-structured approaches to interviewing of value in the field of in-depth child welfare interviews? Do they have the same beneficial effects on the content and style of interview practice that have been demonstrated for the setting of investigative interviews (Orbach et al, 2000)?

Methods of safely reducing the numbers of uncertain or inconclusive outcomes from in-depth or forensic interviews are an important area for further research and practice development. The extended forensic evaluation model (Carnes et al, 1999) provides a structured approach to extending in-depth assessments over several sessions without repetition or inappropriate suggestion. The aim is to create an atmosphere of trust between practitioner and child, without coercion or undue influence. The authors found that, generally, an eight-session model was needed in order to achieve this aim.

As stressed in the section on training, above, it remains an empirical question as to whether a programme of continuing peer audit and review of practice does in fact achieve the desired goal of better quality and more effective interviews.

Hopefully, by the time this book is due for revision, there will have been advances in some of these areas of practice and in other, as yet unseen, areas in this work. As has been repeated throughout this book, the stakes for children who wish to communicate adverse events and experiences of victimisation are so high that to fail them – through false negative or false positive findings, or through prolonged indecision and uncertainty – is a travesty that practitioners in the field continue to strive to overcome.

# References

ABCD Consortium (1993) *Abuse and Children Who Are Disabled (ABCD) Pack*. Leicester: NSPCC.

Abney, V. (2002) Cultural competency in the field of child maltreatment. In *The APSAC Handbook on Child Maltreatment* (eds J. Myers, L. Berliner, J. Briere, *et al*), pp. 477–486. London: Sage.

Adcock, M. (2001) The core assessment: how to synthesise information and make judgements. In *The Child's World: Assessing Children in Need* (ed. J. Horwath), pp 75–97. London: Jessica Kingsley.

Aldridge, A. & Cameron, S. (1999) Interviewing child witnesses: questioning techniques and the role of training. *Applied Developmental Science*, **3**, 136–147.

Aldridge, M. & Wood, J. (1998) *Interviewing Children: A Guide for Child Care and Forensic Practitioners*. Chichester: Wiley.

Anderson, J. C., Martin, J. L., Mullen, P. E., *et al* (1993) The prevalence of childhood sexual abuse experiences in a community sample of women. *Journal of the American Academy of Child and Adolescence Psychiatry*, **32**, 911–919.

Angold, A. (1994) Clinical interviewing with children and adolescents. In *Child and Adolescent Psychiatry: Modern Approaches* (3rd edn) (eds M. Rutter, E. Taylor & L. Hersov), pp. 51–63. London: Blackwell Scientific.

— (2000) Assessment in child and adolescent psychiatry. In *New Oxford Textbook of Psychiatry* (eds M. Gelder, J. Lopez-Ibor & N. Andreasen), pp. 1770–1775. Oxford: Oxford University Press.

— (2002) Diagnostic interviews with parents and children. In *Child and Adolescent Psychiatry* (eds M. Rutter & E. Taylor), pp. 32–51. London: Blackwell.

Atkinson, R., Atkinson, R., Smith, E., *et al* (1996) *Hillgard's Introduction to Psychology*. London: Harcourt Brace.

Banks, N. (1999) *White Counsellors – Black Clients: Theory, Research, and Practice*. Aldershot: Ashgate.

Berliner, L. & Barbieri, M. (1984) The testimony of the child victim of sexual assault. *Journal of Social Issues*, **40**, 125–137.

— & Conte, J. (1995) The effects of disclosure and intervention on sexually abused children. *Child Abuse and Neglect*, **19**, 371–384.

Boat, B. & Everson, M. (1988) Use of anatomical dolls among professionals in child sexual abuse evaluations. *Child Abuse and Neglect*, **12**, 171–179.

—, — & Holland, J. (1990) Maternal perceptions of non-abused young childrens' behaviours after the childrens' exposure to anatomical dolls. *Child Welfare*, **69**, 389–400.

Bornstein, M. & Lamb, M. (1992) *Development in Infancy: An Introduction*. London: McGraw-Hill.

Bottoms, B., Goodman, G., Schwartz-Kenney, B., *et al* (2002) Understanding children's use of secrecy in the context of eyewitness reports. *Law and Human Behaviour*, **26**, 285–313.

Bourg, W., Broderick, R., Flagor, R., *et al* (1999) *A Child Interviewer's Guide Book*. London: Sage.

Bradley, A. & Wood, J. (1996) How do children tell? The disclosure process in child sexual abuse. *Child Abuse and Neglect*, **20**, 881–891.

Bruck, M., Ceci, S. J., Francoeur, E., *et al* (1995a) 'I hardly cried when I got my shot!' Influencing childrens' reports about a visit to their pediatritian. *Child Development*, **66**, 193–298.

—, —, —, *et al* (1995b) Anatomically detailed dolls do not facilitate preschoolers' reports of a pediatric examination involving genital touching. *Journal of Experimental Psychology: Applied*, **1**, 95–109.

Bull, R. (1995) Innovative techniques for questioning of child witnesses, especially those who are young and those with learning disability. In *Memory and Testimony in the Child Witness* (eds M. Zaragoza, J. Graham, G. Hall, *et al*), pp. 179–194. London: Sage.

Bussey, K. (1992) Childrens' lying and truthfulness: implications for childrens' testimony. In *Cognitive and Social Factors in Early Deception* (eds S. J. Ceci, M. DeSimone Leichtman & M. Putnick). Hillsdale, NJ: Lawrence Erlbaum.

Butler, S., Gross, J. & Hayne, H. (1995) The effect of drawing on memory performance in young children. *Developmental Psychology*, **31**, 597–608.

Butler-Sloss, E. (1988) *Report of the Inquiry into Child Abuse in Cleveland in 1987.* London: HMSO.

Calam, R., Cox, A., Glasgow, D., *et al* (2000) Assessment and therapy with children: can computers help? *Clinical Psychology and Psychiatry*, **5**, 329–345.

Campis, L., Hebden-Curtis, J. & DeMaso, R. (1993) Developmental differences in detection and disclosure of sexual abuse. *Journal of the American Academy of Child and Adolescent Psychiatry*, **32**, 920–924.

Cantlon, J., Payne, G. & Erbaugh, C. (1996) Outcome based practice: disclosure rates of child sexual abuse comparing allegation blind and allegation informed structured interviews. *Child Abuse and Neglect*, **20**, 1113–1120.

Carnes, C., Wilson, C. & Nelson-Gardell, D. (1999) Extended forensic evaluation when sexual abuse is suspected: a model and preliminary data. *Child Maltreatment*, **4**, 242–254.

Ceci, S. J. & Bruck, M. (1995) *Jeopardy in the Courtroom: A Scientific Analysis of Children's Testimony*. Washington, DC: American Psychological Association.

— & DeSimone Leichtman, M. (1992) 'I know that you know that I know that you broke the toy': a brief report of recursive awareness among 3 year-olds. In *Cognitive and Social Factors in Early Deception* (eds S. J. Ceci, M. DeSimone Leichtman & M. Putnick), pp 1–9. Hillsdale, NJ: Lawrence Erlbaum.

— & Friedman, R. (2000) The suggestibility of children: scientific research and legal implications. *Cornell Law Review*, **86**, 33–108.

—, Huffman, M. C. L., Smith, E., *et al* (1994) Repeatedly thinking about a non-event: source misattributions among preschoolers. *Consciousness and Cognition*, **3**, 388–407.

Cicchetti, D. (1989) How research on child maltreatment has informed the study of child development: perspectives from developmental psychopathology. In *Child Maltreatment: Theory and Research on the Theory and Causes of Child Abuse and Neglect* (eds D. Cicchetti & V. Carlson), pp. 377–431. Cambridge: Cambridge University Press.

— & Toth, S. (1995) A developmental psychopathology perspective on child abuse and neglect. *Journal of the American Academy of Child and Adolescent Psychiatry*, **34**, 541–565.

Clyde, Lord (1992) *The Report of the Enquiry on the Removal of Children from Orkney in February 1991*. London: HMSO.

Conway, M. (1996) Autobiographical knowledge and autobiographical memories. In *Remembering Our Past: Studies in Autobiographical Memory* (ed. D. C. Rubin), pp. 67–93. Cambridge: Cambridge University Press.

Cox, A. (1994) Interviews with parents. In *Child and Adolescent Psychiatry: Modern Approaches* (3rd edn) (eds M. Rutter, E. Taylor & L. Hersov), pp. 34–50. Oxford: Blackwell Science.

Daniel, B., Wassell, S. & Gilligan, R. (1999) *Child Development for Child Protection Workers*. London: Jessica Kingsley.

Jones, D. P. H. (2003) *Communicating with Vulnerable Children*. London: Gaskell.

Davey, R. & Hill, J. (1999) The variability of practice in interviews used by professionals to investigate child sexual abuse. *Child Abuse and Neglect*, **23**, 571–578.

Davies, G. & Westcott, H. (1998) *The Child Witness and the Memorandum of Good Practice: A Research Review*. London: Home Office.

—, Wilson, C., Mitchell, R., *et al* (1995) *Video Taping of Children's Evidence: An Evaluation*. London: Home Office.

—, Marshall, E. & Robertson, N. (1998) *Child Abuse: Training Investigating Officers*. London: Home Office.

de Mello, R. (2000) *Human Rights Act, 1998: A Practical Guide*. London: Jordans.

DeLoache, J. S. (1995) The use of dolls in interviewing young children. In *Memory and Testimony in the Child Witness* (eds M. Zaragoza, J. Graham, G. Hall, *et al*), pp. 160–178. London: Sage.

Department of Health (1989) *An Introduction to the Children Act, 1989*. London: HMSO.

— (1991) *Child Abuse: A Study of Enquiry Reports 1980–1989*. London: HMSO.

— (1994) *The Child, The Court, and The Video: A Study of the Implementation of the Memorandum of Good Practice on Video Interviewing of Child Witnesses*. London: Social Services Inspectorate.

— (1995) *Child Protection: Messages from Research*. London: HMSO.

— (2000) *Assessing Children in Need and Their Families: Practice Guidance*. London: Stationery Office.

— (2001) *Reference Guide to Consent for Examination or Treatment*. London: Department of Health.

—, Home Office & Department for Education and Employment (1999) *Working Together to Safeguard Children: A Guide to Inter-agency Working to Safeguard and Promote the Welfare of Children*. London: Stationery Office.

—, Department for Education and Employment & Home Office (2000) *Framework for the Assessment of Children in Need and Their Families*. London: Stationery Office.

Dickenson, D. & Jones, D. P. H. (1995) True wishes: the philosophy and developmental psychology of children's informed consent. *Philosophy, Psychiatry and Psychology*, **2**, 287–303.

Dutt, R. & Phillips, M. (2000) Assessing black children in need and their families. In *Assessing Children in Need and Their Families: Practice Guidance* (ed. Department of Health), pp. 37–72. London: Stationery Office.

Endres, J., Poggenpohl, C. & Erben, C. (1999) Repetitions, warnings, and video: cognitive and motivation components in pre-school children's suggestibility. *Legal and Criminological Psychology*, **4**, 129–146.

Everson, M. & Boat, B. (1994) Putting the anatomical doll controversy in perspective: an examination of the major uses and criticisms of the dolls in child sexual abuse evaluations. *Child Abuse and Neglect*, **18**, 113–129.

Faller, K. (1984) Is the child victim of sexual abuse telling the truth? *Child Abuse and Neglect*, **8**, 473–481.

Farmer, E. & Owen, M. (1995) *Child Protection Practice: Private Risks and Public Remedies*. London: HMSO.

Fergusson, D. M. & Mullen, P. E. (1999) *Child Sexual Abuse: An Evidence Based Perspective*. London: Sage.

Finkelhor, D. (1984) *Child Sexual Abuse: New Theory & Research*. London: Macmillan.

— (1994) Current information on the scope and nature of child sexual abuse. *Future of Children*, **4**, 31–53.

— & Kendall-Tackett, K. (1997) The developmental perspective on the childhood impact of crime, abuse, and violent victimisation. In *Developmental Perspectives on Trauma: Theory, Research and Intervention* (eds D. Cicchetti & S. Toth), pp. 1–32. New York: University of Rochester Press.

Fleming, J. M. (1997) Prevalence of childhood sexual abuse in a community sample of Australian women. *Medical Journal of Australia*, **166**, 65–68.

Freeman, K. & Morris, T. (1999) Investigative interviewing with children: evaluation of the effectiveness of the training programme for child protective service workers. *Child Abuse and Neglect*, **23**, 701–713.

Gathercole, S. (1998) The development of memory. *Journal of Child Psychology and Psychiatry*, **39**, 3–27.

Gee, S., Gregory, M. & Pipe, M. (1999) 'What colour is your pet dinosaur?' The impact of pre-interview training and question type on children's answers. *Legal and Criminological Psychology*, **4**, 111–128.

Gibbons, J., Conroy, S. & Bell, C. (1995). *Operating the Child Protection System: A Study of Child Protection Practices in English Local Authorities*. London: HMSO.

Goodman, G., Batterman-Faunce, J., Schaaf, J., *et al* (2002) Nearly four years after an event: children's eye witness memory and adults' perceptions of children's accuracy. *Child Abuse and Neglect*, **26**, 849–884.

—, Pyle, L., Jones, D. P. H., *et al* (1992) Testifying in court: emotional effects of criminal court testimony on child sexual assault victims. *Monographs of the Society for Research in Child Development*, **57** (5, Serial No. 229), 1–161.

Goodman, R. & Scott, S. (1997) Assessment. In *Child Psychiatry*, ch. 1, especially pp. 13–17. Oxford: Blackwell Science.

Goodman-Brown, T., Edelstein, R., Goodman, G., *et al* (2003) Why children tell: a model of children's disclosure of sexual abuse. *Child Abuse and Neglect*, **27**, in press.

Goodyer, I. (1991) *Life Events, Development and Childhood Psychopathology*. Chichester: Wiley.

Gough, D., Boddy, F., Dunning, N., *et al* (1993) *The Management of Child Abuse: A Longitudinal Study of Child Abuse in Glasgow*, Central Research Unit paper. Edinburgh: Scottish Office.

Graham, P., Turk, J. & Verhulst, F. (1999) Introduction. In *Child Psychiatry: A Developmental Approach*, ch. 1, especially pp. 25–33. Oxford: Oxford University Press.

Greenstock, J. & Pipe, M. (1996) Interviewing children about past events: the influence of peer support and misleading questions. *Child Abuse and Neglect*, **20**, 69–80.

Hallett, C. & Birchall, E. (1992) *Co-ordination in Child Protection*. London: HMSO.

Hamby, S. & Finkelhor, D. (2000) The victimisation of children: recommendations for assessment and instrument development. *Journal of the American Academy of Child and Adolescent Psychiatry*, **39**, 829–840.

Hargie, O. & Tourish, D. (1999) The psychology of interpersonal skill. In *Handbook of the Psychology of Interviewing* (eds A. Memon & R. Bull), pp. 71–87. Chichester: Wiley.

Heiman, M. (1992) Putting the puzzle together: validating allegations of child sexual abuse. *Journal of Child Psychology and Psychiatry*, **33**, 311–329.

Hendry, E. & Jones, J. (1997) Dilemmas and opportunities in training around the Memorandum. In *Perspectives on the Memorandum: Policy, Practice, and Research in Investigative Interviewing* (eds H. Westcott & J. Jones), pp. 141–153. Aldershot: Arena.

Hershkowitz, I. (2001) A case study of child sexual false allegation. *Child Abuse and Neglect*, **25**, 1397–1411.

Hindley, P. & Brown, R. (1994) Psychiatric aspects of specific sensory impairments. In *Child and Adolescent Psychiatry: Modern Approaches* (eds M. Rutter, E. Taylor & L. Hersov), pp. 720–736. Oxford: Blackwell Science.

Home Office & Department of Health (1992) *Memorandum of Good Practice on Video Recorded Interviews with Child Witnesses in Criminal Proceedings*. London: HMSO.

—, Lord Chancellor's Department, Crown Prosecution Service, *et al* (2002) *Achieving Best Evidence in Criminal Proceedings: Guidance for Vulnerable or Intimidated Witnesses, Including Children*. London: Home Office.

Horowitz, S., Lamb, M., Esplin, P., *et al* (1995) Establishing ground truth in studies of child sexual abuse. *Expert Evidence*, **4**, 42–51.

Howe, M. & Courage, M. (1997) The emergence and early development of autobiographical memory. *Psychological Review*, **104**, 499–523.

Howlin, P. & Clements, J. (1994) Is it possible to assess the impact of abuse on children with pervasive developmental disorders? *Journal of Autism and Developmental Disorders*, **25**, 337–354.

— & Jones, D. P. H. (1996) An assessment approach to abuse allegations made through facilitated communication. *Child Abuse and Neglect*, **20**, 103–110.

Hudson, B. (2000) Interagency collaboration – a sceptical view. In *Critical Practice in Health and Social Care* (eds A. Brechin, H. Brown & M. Eby), pp 253–274. London: Open University/Sage.

Jones, D. P. H. (1992) *Interviewing the Sexually Abused Child: Investigation of Suspected Abuse* (4th edn). London: Gaskell.

— (1994) Autism, facilitated communication and allegations of child abuse and neglect. *Child Abuse and Neglect*, **18**, 491–493.

— (1996) Editorial. Gradual disclosure by sexual assault victims – a sacred cow? *Child Abuse and Neglect*, **20**, 879–880.

— (1997) Assessment of suspected child sexual abuse. In *The Battered Child* (5th edn) (eds R. Helfer, R. Kempe & R. Krugman), pp. 296–312. Chicago: University of Chicago Press.

— (1999) Editorial. Training for investigative interviews with children. *Child Abuse and Neglect*, **23**, 699–700.

— (2000a) Editorial. Disclosure of child sexual abuse. *Child Abuse and Neglect*, **24**, 269–271.

— (2000b) Child abuse and neglect. In *The New Oxford Textbook of Psychiatry* (eds M. Gelder, J. Lopez-Ibor & N. Andreasen), pp. 1825–1834. Oxford: Oxford University Press.

— & McGraw, J. M. (1987) Reliable and fictitious accounts of sexual abuse to children. *Journal of Interpersonal Violence*, **2**, 27–45.

— & Seig, A. (1988) Child sexual abuse allegations in custody or visitation disputes. In *Sexual Abuse Allegations in Custody and Visitation Disputes* (eds B. Nicholson & J. Buckley). Washington, DC: American Bar Association.

— & Ramchandani, P. (1999) *Child Sexual Abuse – Informing Practice from Research.* Oxford: Radcliffe Medical Press.

—, Dickenson, D. & Devereux, J. (1994) The favoured child. *Journal of Medical Ethics*, **20**, 108–111.

Jouriles, E., Norwood, W., McDonald, R., *et al* (2001) Domestic violence and child adjustment. In *Interparental Conflict and Child Development: Theory, Research and Applications* (eds J. Grych & F. Fincham), pp. 315–336. Cambridge: Cambridge University Press.

JRF, Triangle & NSPCC (2001) *'Two Way Street': Training Video and Handbook About Communicating with Disabled Children and Young People.* Leicester: NSPCC.

Kennedy, M. (1992a) Not the only way to communicate: a challenge to voice in child protection work. *Child Abuse Review*, **1**, 169–177.

— (1992b) Children with severe disabilities: too many assumptions. *Child Abuse Review*, **1**, 185–187.

— (1993) Human aids to communication. In *Abuse and Children Who Are Disabled, Reader and Resource Pack* (ed. ABCD Consortium), pp. 88–102. Leicester: NSPCC.

Kolko, D. (2002) Child Physical Abuse. In *The APSAC Handbook on Child Maltreatment* (eds J. Myers, L. Berliner, J. Briere, *et al*) pp. 21–44. London: Sage.

—, Kazdin, A. & Day, B. (1996) Children's perspectives in the assessment of family violence: psychometric characteristics and comparison parents' report. *Child Maltreatment*, **1**, 165–167.

Kolvin, I., Steiner, H., Bamford, F., *et al* (Independent Second Opinion Panel, Northern Regional Health Authority) (1988) Child sexual abuse – some principles of good practice. *British Journal of Hospital Medicine*, **39**, 54–62.

Lamb, M., Herskowitz, I., Sternberg, K., *et al* (1996) Investigative interviews of alleged sexual abuse victims with and without anatomical dolls. *Child Abuse and Neglect*, **20**, 1251–1259.

—, Sternberg, K. & Esplin, P. (1998) Conducting investigative interviews of alleged sexual abuse victims. *Child Abuse and Neglect*, **22**, 813–823.

—, —, Orbach, Y., *et al* (1999) Forensic interviews of children. In *Handbook of the Psychology of Interviewing* (eds A. Memon & R. Bull), pp. 253–278. Chichester: Wiley.

Laming, H. (2003) *The Victoria Climbie Inquiry*. London: Stationery Office.

Lanktree, C., Briere, J. & Zaidi, L. (1991) Incidence and impact of sexual abuse in a child out-patient sample: the role of direct enquiry. *Child Abuse and Neglect*, 15, 447–454.

Lawson, L. & Chaffin, M. (1992) False negatives in sexual abuse disclosure interviews. *Journal of Interpersonal Violence*, 7, 532–542.

Leichtman, M. D. & Ceci, S. J. (1995) The effects of stereotypes and suggestions on preschoolers' reports. *Developmental Psychology*, **31**, 568–578.

Lindsay, D. S. (2002) Children's source monitoring. In *Children's Testimony: A Handbook of Psychological Research and Forensic Practice* (eds H. Westcott, G. Davies & R. Bull), pp. 83–98. Chichester: Wiley.

Macfie, J., Cicchetti, D. & Toth, S. (2001) Dissociation in maltreated versus non-maltreated pre-school-aged children. *Child Abuse and Neglect*, **25**, 1253–1267.

MacIntyre, D. & Carr, A. (1999) Helping children to the other side of silence: the study of the impact of the 'Stay Safe' programme on Irish children's disclosures of sexual victimisation. *Child Abuse and Neglect*, **23**, 1327–1340.

Macpherson, W. (1999) *The Stephen Lawrence Enquiry*. London: Stationery Office.

Madonna, P., Van Scoyk, S. & Jones, D. P. H. (1991) Family interactions within incest and non-incest families. *American Journal of Psychiatry*, **148**, 46–49.

Marchant, R. & Jones, M. (2000) Assessing the needs of disabled children and their families. In *Assessing Children in Need and Their Families: Practice Guidance* (ed. Department of Health), pp. 73–112. London: Stationery Office.

— & Page, M. (1992) Bridging the gap: investigating the abuse of children with multiple disabilities. *Child Abuse Review*, **1**, 179–183.

— & — (1997) The Memorandum and disabled children. In *Perspectives on the Memorandum: Policy, Practice, and Research in Investigative Interviewing* (eds H. Westcott & J. Jones), pp. 67–79. Aldershot: Arena.

Masten, A. & Coatsworth, J. (1998) The development of competence in favourable and unfavourable environments: lessons from research on successful children. *American Psychologist*, 53, 205–220.

McGough, L. S. (1996) Coventry: achieving real reform – the case for American interviewing protocols. *Monographs of the Society for Research in Child Development*, **61** (4–5, no. 248), 188–203.

Memon, A. (1998) Telling it all: the cognitive interview. In *Psychology and Law: Truthfulness, Accuracy and Credibility* (eds A. Memon, A. Vrij & R. Bull), pp. 170–187. London: McGraw-Hill.

Mezey, G. & Robbins, I. (2000) The impact of criminal victimisation. In *New Oxford Textbook of Psychiatry* (eds M. Gelder, J. Lopez-Ibor & N. Andreasen), pp. 2083–2088. Oxford: Oxford University Press.

Mian, M., Wehrspann, W., Klajner-Diamond, H., *et al* (1986) Review of 125 children six years of age and under who were sexually abused. *Child Abuse and Neglect*, **10**, 223–229.

Milne, R. (1999) Interviewing children with learning disabilities. In *Handbook of the Psychology of Interviewing* (eds A. Memon & R. Bull), pp. 165–180. Chichester: Wiley.

Jones, D. P. H. (2003) *Communicating with Vulnerable Children*. London: Gaskell.

— & Bull, R. (1996) Interviewing children with mild learning disability with the cognitive interview. In *Investigative and Forensic Decision Making: Issues in Criminological Psychology* (eds N. K. Clark & G. M. Stephenson), pp 44–51. Leicester: British Psychological Society.

Morrison, J. & Anders, T. (1999) *Interviewing Children and Adolescents: Skills and Strategies for Effective DSM–IV Diagnosis*. London: Guilford Press.

Mortimer, A. & Shepherd, E. (1999) Frames of mind: schemata guiding cognition and conduct in the interviewing of suspected offenders. In *Handbook of the Psychology of Interviewing* (eds A. Memon & R. Bull), pp. 293–315. Chichester: Wiley.

Moston, S. & Egleberg, T. (1992) The effects of social support on children's eye witness testimony. *Applied Cognitive Psychology*, **6**, 61–75.

Mulder, M. & Vrij, A. (1996) Explaining conversational rules to children: an intervention study to facilitate children's accurate responses. *Child Abuse and Neglect*, **20**, 623–631.

Mussen, P., Conger, J., Kagan, J., *et al* (1990) *Child Development and Personality*. New York: Harper Collins

National Assembly for Wales (2000) *Working Together to Safeguard Children: A Guide to Inter-Agency Working to Safeguard and Promote the Welfare of Children*. London: Stationery Office.

— (2001) *Framework for the Assessment of Children in Need and their Families*. London: Stationery Office.

National Center on Child Abuse and Neglect (NCCAN) (1988) *Study of National Incidence and Prevalence of Child Abuse and Neglect: 1988*. Washington, DC: US Department of Health and Human Services.

NSPCC/Chailey Heritage (1998) *Turning Points: A Resource Pack for Communicating with Children*. London: NSPCC.

Oates, R. K., Jones, D. P. H., Denson, D., *et al* (2000) Erroneous concerns about child sexual abuse. *Child Abuse and Neglect*, **24**, 149–157.

Orbach, Y. & Lamb, M. (2000) Enhancing children's narratives in investigative interviews. *Child Abuse and Neglect*, **24**, 1631–1648.

—, Hershkowitz, I., Lamb, M., *et al* (2000) Assessing the value of scripted protocols for forensic interviews of alleged abuse victims. *Child Abuse and Neglect*, **24**, 733–752.

Pezdek, K. & Hinz, T. (2002) The construction of false events in memory. In *Children's Testimony: A Handbook of Psychological Research and Forensic Practice* (eds H. Westcott, G. Davies & R. Bull), pp. 99–116. Chichester: Wiley.

Phillips, M. (1993) Investigative interviewing – issues of race and culture. In *Investigative Interviewing with Children – Trainer's Pack*, pp. 50–55. Milton Keynes: Open University Press.

Pipe, M. E., Salmon, K. & Priestley, G. (2002) Enhancing children's accounts: how useful are non-verbal techniques? In *Children's Testimony: A Handbook of Psychological Research and Forensic Practice* (eds H. Westcott, G. Davies & R. Bull), pp. 161–174. London: Wiley.

Poole, D. & Lamb, M. (1998) *Investigative Interviews of Children: A Guide for Helping Professionals*. Washington, DC: American Psychological Association.

Poole, D. A. & Lindsay, D. (1998) Assessing the accuracy of children's reports: lessons from the investigations of child sexual abuse. *Applied and Preventative Psychology*, **7**, 1–26.

Porter, S., Yuille, J. & Bent, A. (1995) A comparison of the eye-witness accounts of deaf and hearing children. *Child Abuse and Neglect*, **19**, 51–61.

Powell, M. & Thomson, D. (1997) The effect of an intervening interview on children's ability to remember an occurrence of a repeated event. *Legal and Criminological Psychology*, **2**, 247–262.

Prescott, A., Bank, L., Reid, J., *et al* (2000) The veridicality of punitive childhood experiences reported by adolescents and young adults. *Child Abuse and Neglect*, **24**, 411–423.

Prior, V., Lynch, M. & Glaser, D. (1994) *Messages from Children: Children's Evaluation of the Professional's Response to Child Sexual Abuse.* London: NCH Action for Children.

Putnam, F. (1997) *Dissociation in Children and Adolescents: A Developmental Perspective.* New York: Guilford Press.

*Re H* (Children Care Proceedings Section – Abuse) (2000) *Family Court Reports,* **2**, 499–511.

Roberts, J. & Taylor, C. (1993) Sexually abused children speak out. In *Child Abuse and Child Abusers* (ed. L. Waterhouse), pp. 13–37. London: Jessica Kingsley.

Salmon, K. (2001) Remembering and reporting by children: the influence of cues and props. *Clinical Psychology Review,* **21**, 267–300.

Sauzier, M. (1989) Disclosure of child sexual abuse: for better or for worse. *Psychiatric Clinics of North America,* **12**, 455–469.

Saywitz, K. (1995) Improving children's testimony: the question, the answer, and the environment. In *Memory and Testimony in the Child Witness* (eds M. Zaragaza, J. Graham, G. Hall, *et al*), pp. 113–140. London: Sage.

—— & Snyder, L. (1993) Improving children's testimony with preparation. In *Child Victims, Child Witnesses: Understanding and Improving Testimony* (eds G. Goodman & B. Bottoms), pp. 117–146. London: Guilford Press.

——, Goodman, G., Nicholas, E. & Moan, S. (1991) Children's memories of a physical examination involving genital touch: implications for reports of child sexual abuse. *Journal of Consulting and Clinical Psychology,* **59**, 682–691.

Sgroi, M., Porter, F. & Blick, L. (1982) Validation of child sexual abuse. In *Handbook of Clinical Intervention in Child Sexual Abuse* (ed. S. M. Sgroi), pp. 39–79. Lexington, MA: D. C. Heath.

Sharland, E., Seal, H., Croucher, M., *et al* (1996) *Professional Intervention in Child Sexual Abuse.* London: HMSO.

Shemmings, D. (1998) *In on the Act: Involving Children in Family Support and Child Protection – A Training Pack for Professionals.* Norwich: University of East Anglia.

—— (ed.) (1999) *Involving Children in Family Support and Child Protection.* London: Stationery Office.

Siegel, D. (2001) Memory: an overview, with emphasis on developmental, interpersonal, and neurobiological aspects. *Journal of the American Academy of Child and Adolescent Psychiatry,* **40**, 997–1011.

Smith, D., Letourneau, E., Saunders, B., *et al* (2000) Delay in disclosure in childhood rape: results from a national survey. *Child Abuse and Neglect,* **24**, 273–287.

Sternberg, K., Lamb, M., Hershkowitz, I., *et al* (1997) Effects of introductory style on children's abilities to describe experiences of sexual abuse. *Child Abuse and Neglect,* **21**, 1133–1146.

——, ——, Davies, G., *et al* (2001) Memorandum of good practice: theory versus application. *Child Abuse and Neglect,* **25**, 669–681.

Summit, R. (1983) The child's sexual abuse accommodation syndrome. *Child Abuse and Neglect,* **7**, 177–193.

Tan, J. & Jones, D. P. H. (2001) Children's consent. *Current Opinion in Psychiatry,* **14**, 303–307.

Vrij, A. (2002) Deception in children: literature review and implications for children's testimony. In *Children's Testimony: A Handbook of Psychological Research and Forensic Practice* (eds H. Westcott, G. Davies and R. Bull), pp. 175–194. Chichester Wiley.

Wade, A. & Westcott, H. (1997) No easy answers: children's perspectives on investigative interviews. In *Perspectives on the Memorandum* (eds H. Westcott & J. Jones), pp. 51–65. Aldershot: Arena.

Wade, D. (1998) *Measurement in Neurological Rehabilitation.* Oxford: Oxford University Press.

Walker, A. G. (1994) *Handbook on Questioning Children: A Linguistic Perspective.* Washington, DC: American Bar Association.

Jones, D. P. H. (2003) *Communicating with Vulnerable Children.* London: Gaskell.

Walker, N. & Hunt, J. (1998) Interviewing child victim-witnesses: how you ask is what you get. In *Eyewitness Memory: Theoretical and Applied Perspectives* (eds C. Thompson, D. Herrmann, J. Read, *et al*), pp. 55–87. Mahwah, NJ: Erlbaum.

Warner, J. & Hansen, D. (1997) Identification and reporting of child abuse by medical professionals: a critical review. *Child Abuse and Neglect*, **18**, 11–25.

Warren, A., Woodall, C., Hunt, J. & Perry, N. (1996) 'It sounds good in theory, but...': two investigative interviewers follow guidelines based on memory research? *Child Maltreatment*, **1**, 231–245.

Wattam, C. (1992) *Making a Case in Child Protection*. Chichester: Wiley.

Westcott, H. & Davies, G. (1996). Sexually abused children's and young people's perspectives on investigative interview. *British Journal of Social Work*, **26**, 451–474.

—, — & Bull, R. (2002) *Children's Testimony: A Handbook of Psychological Research and Forensic Ppractice*. Chichester: Wiley.

— & Jones, D. P. H. (1999) Annotation. The abuse of disabled children. *Journal of Child Psychology and Psychiatry*, **40**, 497–506.

— & Jones, D. P. H. (2003) Are children reliable witnesses to their experiences? In *Studies in the Assessment of Parenting* (eds P. Reder, S. Duncan & C. Lucey). London: Routledge.

Wheeler, M., Stuss, D. & Tulving, E. (1997) Towards a theory of episodic memory: frontal lobes and autonoetic consciousness. *Psychological Bulletin*, **121**, 331–354.

White, T. L., Leichtman, M. D. & Ceci, S. J. (1997) The good, the bad and the ugly: accuracy, inaccuracy and elaboration in preschoolers' reports about a past event. *Applied Cognitive Psychology*, **11**, S37–S54.

Wood, J., McClure, K. & Birch, R. (1996) Suggestions for improving interviews in child protection agencies. *Child Maltreatment*, **1**, 223–230.

World Health Organization (1980) *International Classification of Impairment, Disabilities and Handicaps*. Geneva: World Health Organization.

Yarrow, L. (1960) Interviewing children. In *Handbook of Research Methods in Child Development* (ed. P. Mussen), pp. 561–602. New York: Wiley.

Jones, D. P. H. (2003) *Communicating with Vulnerable Children*. London: Gaskell.

**181**

# Index

## Compiled by Linda English

accuracy of accounts 1–2, 117–120, 163–169
ADHD (attention-deficit hyperactivity disorder) 44–45
adolescents 30–31, 109, 131, 143
adult recollections of abuse 79–80
adversity, effects on children 38–43
aggressive behaviour 98–99, 135, 145
ambiguous words 27
anatomical drawings 155
anatomically detailed dolls 145, 150, 153–154
anxiety 42, 45, 46
'any', use of 27
attachment 9, 30, 41, 76, 119
attention seeking 44
audio-recording 128–129
augmentative communications systems 59–60
authority effects 19, 25, 126
autism 60, 111
autobiographical memory 11, 12–13, 14–16

behaviour, observation of 145–147
behaviour change 98–99, 132, 134–135
behaviour problems 41, 42, 43–44, 45, 135, 167
bias among practitioners 47, 68–70, 96–97, 163
bilingual children 23, 53, 54
black children 49–50, 51–52
blind interviews 120–121
boundaries of intimate care 76
bullying 138

'Can you...?' questions 28
carers, advice for 157–161

case examples 4–5, 24, 91–92, 98–99
child and adolescent mental health 102, 104
child as expert 20, 22, 25, 105, 106
Children Act 1989: 107
    Section 17: 112
    Section 47: 3, 4, 88, 106, 112, 114
children in need 88, 102, 107–108
child sexual abuse see sexual abuse
coercive interviewing 70
cognitive interview 60
communication aids 59–60
communication impairments 23, 55, 76, 137, 148
comparisons, questions about 27
complex language, avoidance of 22, 26–27, 29
confidentiality 94, 109, 125, 143
consent 94
consistency of recall over time 19–22, 167–168
continuing professional development 162, 171
conversational style 22, 25
coping strategies 39, 40
core assessments 112, 113, 114, 115
core skills and basic principles 64–72
    awareness of entire transaction 67
    capacity to listen 65–66
    capacity to manage assessment 66–67
    emotional warmth 66
    empathy 66
    and first responses to children's concerns 95–97
    genuine interest 66
    implications for practitioner 71
    positive professional qualities 71–72
    qualities to avoid 72
    respect 66

Jones, D. P. H. (2003) *Communicating with Vulnerable Children*. London: Gaskell.

**183**

self-management 67–69
  technique 69–70
  understanding 66
criminal offences 4, 5, 78, 88, 106, 113,
  140–141
cultural identity 51
cultural issues 30, 49–55, 109–110
cultural racism 51
culture, defined 51

deaf children 57–59
deception by children 36–37
declarative memory 11
depression 42, 45
developmental issues 9–32, 39, 41–42,
  75–76, 165
disabled children 23, 55–63
  black 49
  communication aids 59–60
  disability defined 56
  implications for practitioners 60–63
  importance of disability for practitioners
    56
  initial assessments 109, 110
  and play 148
  sensory impairment 57–59
  social model of disability 55–56
  World Health Organization classification
    56
discipline, questions about 110
disclosure 73–83
  adult recollections of abuse 79–80
  advice for concerned parents 157–159
  after discovery of physical harm 79
  assessing accuracy of child's account
    167–168
  delay in 80–81, 82–83
  developmental considerations 75–76
  first responses to children's concerns
    95–96
  impact of sexual assault prevention
    programmes 81
  numbers in child protection system
    77–78
  presentations of sexual abuse allegations
    78–79
  social and emotional factors 76–77
  studies of children's experiences 79
  use and misuse of term 73–74
disclosure interview 74
discrimination 49, 50, 55–56
dissociation 42, 45

diversity and difference 49–63
doctors 98
documentation of conversations 29, 99,
  113, 128–129
dolls 151
  anatomically detailed 145, 150, 153–154
  purposes of use 148, 149
  as representations 150, 154
domestic violence 5, 40, 41, 134, 138
'don't know' answers 126
drawings 147–149, 150–151, 152–153,
  155
dual heritage 51

echolalia 57
educational services, first assessments by
  102–103, 112
embarrassment 76, 77, 152
emotional abuse 35
emotional development 30–31
emotional distress
  in child after interview 143
  in parents 123, 157, 159
emotional factors, and disclosure 76–77
emotional problems 41, 42, 45–46, 167
emotional warmth 66
empathy 66
encoding 13–14
encouragement cues 70
environmental reinstatement 148
episodic memory 12, 13
erroneous concerns and cases 33–37
  consequences 34
  errors of commission/omission 69, 71,
    154, 155
  frequency of types of false positives
    34–36
  from adults 35, 37
  from children 35, 36–37
  implications for practitioners 37
  and interviewer bias 69, 96–97
  mechanisms leading to false positives
    36–37
  terminology used 33–34
  and uncommunicative children 47
  and use of screening questions 104–105
ethnicity
  defined 51
  of interviewers 54
ethnic minorities 49–55, 109–110
event memory 11, 142
expectancy (confirmatory bias) 68

Jones, D. P. H. (2003) *Communicating with Vulnerable Children*. London: Gaskell.

expressed emotion 67, 69, 70, 166
eye contact 45, 46, 152

false allegations 33–34
false negative errors 33, 37
false positive errors 33, 34–37, 71
family, information about 54, 110, 168–169
family violence 40
fearfulness 41, 42, 45
first assessments 101, 102–103, 104–105, 112
first responses to children's concerns 91–100
    confidentiality 94
    consent 94
    implications for practitioners 97–100
    policy and procedural issues 92–94
    research findings 95–97
    and training 169–170
five critical components 87, 102
free recall 14, 17

gender of practitioner 44, 54
government guidance 4, 101, 107, 114, 115
grammar 24
group identification 51

handicap 56
health services, first assessments by 102–103, 112
hearing-impaired children 57–59
'How many times...?' questions 28
hyperactive children 44–45

identity concept 51
identity of individuals, questions about 27, 29, 142
impairment(s)
    communication 23, 55, 76, 137, 148
    defined 56
    psychological, resulting from abuse 40
    sensory 57–59
    see also disabled children
inconclusive concerns 35
in-depth interviews 88, 114–144
    advance planning 120–123
    advice for parents/carers before 159–160
    clarification of details 141–142
    closing of interview 143–144
    concerns allayed 140
    concerns confirmed 140–141

direct questions 137–139
duration of sessions 117
ending in uncertainty 139–140, 160–161, 172
enquiry into suspected adverse experiences 132–139
extended forensic evaluation model 172
further exploration 139–142
future directions for practice development 171–172
introductory, rapport-gaining phase 124–127, 130–132
obtaining accurate and useful accounts 117–120
place of indirect, creative approaches 127, 137, 152
policy and procedural context 114–116
preparation of child 123–124
presence of parents 118–119
by professionals other than social workers 116
recording interviews 128–129
research findings and practice implications 116–130
schema for 130–144
specific objectives 121
structure 127–128
and training 170–171
indirect and non-verbal approaches 145–156
    congruence of verbal/non-verbal communications 145, 147
    distinction between observation and interpretation 145–147
    and errors/inaccurate information 148, 149–150, 151, 154, 155
    implications for practitioners 151–155
    in in-depth interviewing 127, 137, 152
    linking toys to specific events 150
    observation of behaviour 145–147
    props 148, 149–150, 153
    research findings 149–151
    and suggestion 148, 151, 153, 155
    and theoretical stances 145
    toys and drawings 147–155
individual differences between children 23, 32, 66
individual identity 51
individual racism 51
information analysis, framework for 162–169
    child's account 164–167
    child's behaviour and emotional state 167
    disclosure process 167–168
    information from family history/ assessment 168–169

medical evidence 169
physiological measures 169
prior accounts/expressions of concern 168
witness statements 168
inhibition of responses 30–31, 76
initial assessments 88, 101–113
    advice for parents/carers after 159–160
    aims 101–102
    choice of question and approach 105–106
    exploratory questions 111
    implications for practitioners 108–111
    policy and procedural context 101–104
    process and decision making 106–108
    professional qualities needed 71–72
    research findings 104–108
institutional racism 51, 52
intelligence 23
intelligibility of child's communications 24
interpreters 53, 58, 59
interviewers see practitioners
investigative interviews 105–106, 107,
    113, 140–141

language development 22–30
    and assessing accuracy of child's account
        165
    and communications which may lead to
        misunderstandings 25–28
    and conversational style 25
    detection of/coping with
        misunderstandings 25
    differences between adults and children
        23–25
    and disclosure 75–76
    grammar and vocabulary 24
    implications for practitioners 28–30
    individual differences 23
    and intelligibility 24
    and sensory impairment 57–58
language differences 23, 52–53, 54
leading questions 14, 18, 72
learning disabilities 44, 55, 57, 60, 76,
    102, 159
listening capacity 65–66, 97
long-term memory 12
lying 36–37

medical evidence 79, 132, 134, 169
memory 10–22
    autobiographical 11, 12–13, 14–16
    declarative 11

defined 11
and disclosure 76
encoding 13–14
episodic 12, 13
event memory 11, 142
implications for practitioners 17
long-term/permanent 12
procedural 11
retrieval 13–14, 15, 16, 17, 60, 148
script memory 15, 16
semantic 12
sensory 11, 12
short-term/working memory 12
source-monitoring difficulties 13,
    15–16, 19
stages 13–14
status 14
storage 13–14
and stress 13, 16
and suggestibility 16, 18–19
mental health problems 40–46
meta-perception 67
minority groups 49–55
misunderstandings
    children's ability to detect/cope with 25
    communications which may lead to 25–30
    and cultural differences 52–53
moral development 31
multi-disciplinary working 93, 107–108, 141
multi-sensory impairment 57

negative term insertion questions 22
neglect 35, 69
neutral subjects, practice with 126, 130–131
non-judgemental approach 47–48
non-verbal communication see indirect and
    non-verbal approaches

object cues (props) 148, 149–150, 153
observation 145–147

parents 157–161
    advice during assessment process 159–160
    advice for first concerns 157–159
    advice when uncertainty persists 160–161
    consent 94
    emotional distress 123, 157, 159
    involvement in initial assessments 108–109
    presence at in-depth interviews 118–119
passive voice, avoidance of 27

pathology 56
peer relationships 9, 30
physical abuse 35, 79, 138, 166, 169
physical disability 55
physical disease/change 79, 132, 134, 169
physical reassurance 42
physiological measures of truthfulness 169
play materials 145, 147–149
  and clarification of details 153, 154
  and cultural differences 55
  to demonstrate 149
  to direct attention to area of interest 148
  to encourage enactment 149
  to encourage rapport 148
  implications for practitioners 151–155
  indirect benefits of use 151
  to label objects/parts of body 148, 154, 155
  and symbolic representation 150, 151, 154
polygraph examination 169
post-traumatic stress disorder (PTSD) 42–43, 45, 46, 52
practitioners
  bias in 47, 68–70, 96–97, 163
  conversational style 22, 25
  core skills and qualities needed 64–72, 95–96
  erroneous concerns by 35
  non-verbal communication 48, 147
  objectivity 108
  personal experience of abuse 67
  positive qualities 71–72
  qualities to avoid 72
  responses to individual interviewers 46, 96
  support/advice from other colleagues 98
  training 32, 68, 93, 169–171
preparation of child
  for in-depth interview 123–124, 160
  for investigative interview 105–106
prepositions 27
pressurising of child 70, 137, 158
procedural memory 11
professionals see practitioners
pronunciation 24, 29
props 148, 149–150, 153
psychological condition of child 38–48
  and assessing accuracy of child's account 167
  effect on commmunication 43–48
  effects of adverse experiences 38–43

implications for practitioners 41–42, 43–46, 47–48
  reluctant/uncommunicative children 46–48
  special problems 42–43

race
  defined 50–51
  and disclosure 78
racial identity 51
racial issues 49–55, 109–110
racism 50, 51, 52, 54
rapport-gaining phase 46, 47, 124–127, 130–132, 152–153
recall 14
  consistency over repeated interviews 20
  consistency over time 19–22
  implications for practitioners 21–22
  of repeated events 15, 16, 17, 20–21, 141–142
  repeated questions within session 20
  use of play materials 148, 149
recognition remembering 14
record keeping 29, 99, 113, 128–129
referrers' errors 35
refugee children 52
reluctant children 46–48
'Remember' questions 28
repeated events, memories of 15, 16, 17, 20–21, 141–142
respect for individual child 66
retrieval 13–14, 15, 16, 17, 60, 148
rough notes, value of 99, 129

salience of events 13, 14, 17, 21
schemas 15, 16
screening questions 104–105
script memories/knowledge 15, 16, 21, 148
secrets 31, 166–167
Section 47 enquiries 3, 4, 88, 106, 112, 114
selective reinforcement 70
self-blame 39, 42, 43
self-development 9, 30
self-esteem 42
self-harm 42, 45, 103, 135
self management 67–69
semantic memory 12
sensitivity to adult responses 69, 95, 147
sensory impairment 55, 57–59
sensory memory 11, 12

sexual abuse 52
  and accommodation syndrome 80
  adult recollections 79–80
  assessing accuracy of child's account
      163–164, 165, 166, 167, 169
  and boundaries of intimate care 76
  delay in disclosure 80–81
  direct questions about 138
  impact of prevention programmes 81
  medical evidence 169
  presentations of allegations 78–79
  rates of substantiation 34–35, 77–78
  social/emotional factors and disclosure
      76–77
  unique/distinguishing details 165
  use of dolls 145, 151, 154
  use of drawings 155
  use of screening questions 104
  validation 163–164
sexual assault prevention programmes 81
sexualised behaviour 73, 111, 135, 166
short-term memory 12
sign languages 58
small-group peer review 171
social development 30–31
social model of disability 55–56
social services departments
  in-depth interviews by 114–116
  initial assessments by 101–113
social support for child 77, 118
source monitoring difficulties 13, 15–16, 19
speech and language difficulties 23
speech and language therapists 23
stereotyping 54, 68–69
substantiation rates 34–35, 77–78
suggestibility 16, 18–19, 21
support from interviewer 30
support person for child 44–45, 118–119

tag questions 22, 26–27
teachers 97–98

threats 77, 166–167
time, communications about 26
touch, communications about 26
toys 147–150, 151–152, 153
training 32, 68, 93, 169–171
typecasting 68–69

uncommunicative children 46–48
understanding
  developmental changes in 10, 75
  professional capacity for 66
unsubstantiated allegations 34

verbal cues 148
victimisation 38–41
  appraisals of 39
  children who harm others 43, 121
  coping strategies 39
  defined 38
  environmental factors 39
  impact on current developmental status
      39
  implications for practitioners 41–42
  psychological effects on child 38–43
video-recording 125, 128–129
visually impaired children 57
vocabulary 24

welfare 1
'When' questions 26, 28
'WH' questions 22, 28, 29
'Why' questions 28
witness, child as 64–65
witness statements 168
working memory 12
World Health Organization classification,
  and disability 56

Jones, D. P. H. (2003) *Communicating with Vulnerable Children*. London: Gaskell.